Staying Alive

How to improve your health and your healthcare

DR PHIL HAMMOND

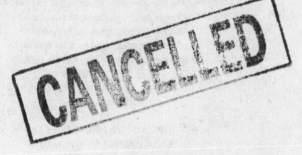

Quercus

First published in 2015 by Quercus.
This edition published in Great Britain in 2019 by Quercus.

Quercus Editions Ltd
Carmelite House
50 Victoria Embankment
London EC4Y 0DZ

An Hachette UK company

A CIP catalogue record for this book is available
from the British Library

PB ISBN 978 1 78747 788 9
Ebook ISBN 978 1 84866 452 4

Every effort has been made to contact copyright holders.
However, the publishers will be glad to rectify in future
editions any inadvertent omissions brought to their attention.

perm... ...ent
...any loss,
...y a
...ok.

Tex... ...n Keynes

...p.A.

CONTENTS

FOREWORD

Health, and a Health Service, for All

In 2018, I toured the UK celebrating 70 years of the NHS and canvassing ideas for a 'People's Plan' to keep the service afloat in the future. The majority of my audience members (admittedly not a random sample) wanted to restore the government's legally binding duty to provide universal healthcare rather than just 'promote' it, which has allowed a whole range of services to be cut or cut back. They were prepared to pay more for health and social care services, but only if the money was spent on supporting frontline services that were proven to work. They preferred the services to be publicly provided, with outsourcing to the private sector only used if the NHS needed help, and only if the providers were 'not for profit' so that any savings went back into the service rather than to shareholders. They wanted longer consultations with staff they knew and who knew them (something that's been proven to improve your care). Above all, they wanted NHS staff to be safe, unstressed and well-rested, and present in sufficient numbers. Most regular users of the NHS observed staff shortages and exhausted doctors and nurses. They wanted legally-mandated safe staffing levels, starting with emergency care and on-call.

There were some funny suggestions too. 'All cabinet members and their families must be treated in the worst performing hospital in the country.' That could drive up standards faster than anything. I also liked 'When people who shelter money in tax havens call an ambulance, it has to come from the Cayman Islands.' There was a strong feeling that tax should be seen as a badge of honour for living in a civilised society rather than money the government grabs off you. If we'd matched the percentage of our GDP that Germany has put into health just since 2000, we'd have put an extra £260 billion into the NHS. Think how fabulous the service could be with that level of investment. A few suggestions were brilliant in their simplicity. 'For one day a year, doctors and patients should tell each other the truth.' And 'Replace hospital beds with bunk beds. Bed crisis sorted.' One of the most popular suggestions was the most unlikely. 'Dr Phil for Health Secretary.'

I have promised to give this my best shot, although I'll somehow have to leapfrog my sitting MP, Jacob Rees-Mogg, first. My philosophy is that 'health for all' should be the political consideration and ambition that overrides all others. Without health – our ability to live a life that we have reason to value – then life itself seems pretty pointless. Health is also our ability to adapt to change and to bounce back when life kicks us in the teeth, something that happens to us all and some much more than others. In this book, I outline CLANGERS as the daily ingredients and joys of health:

Connect
Learn
(BE) **A**ctive
Notice
Give back
Eat well
Relax
Sleep

There is good evidence that each of these habits improves your health, particularly if you get into a routine of doing them at the same time in a 24-hour cycle to fit in with your body's circadian clock (e.g. get up and go to bed at the same time every day, including weekends, aiming for 8 hours of good sleep. Do all your eating in a 12-hour window so your gut has 12 hours off every day. Don't do vigorous exercise for 2 hours before your sleep time, apart from sex).

Good sleep is both the key to health and the key to recovery. The less you sleep, the quicker you die. On the flip side, just about every symptom and illness you have will be improved by better sleep, as will your exercise tolerance, work performance, creativity and diet. I have included sleep tips in this book because they are so important. When I'm health secretary, I'll still be getting 8 hours a night and making sure everyone has a bed to sleep in (around 400,000 children in the UK do not).

As for the NHS, services are so short-staffed and underfunded at present that they simply aren't going to improve radically anytime soon. We are paying the price in all of our public services of choosing to live in a low tax economy. However, there is plenty we could improve on. Many of us are over-medicalised and over-screened, on multiple tablets of minimal benefit and at high risk of side effects when lifestyle medicine through CLANGERS would be far cheaper, more effective, safer and a lot more fun. And your best hope of surviving and thriving with an illness, both in and out of the NHS, also comes down to CLANGERS:

• **CONNECT** with the team treating you, and get to know them as much as you can. Try to see the same person for the same problem. Continuity of care gets the best results.

• **LEARN** as much as you can about your illness, what you can do for yourself to aid recovery, your treatment options, what you are entitled to, the standards of care you should be getting and who to speak to if you have concerns.

• **BE ACTIVE,** both in the management of your illness and preventing further illness. Be your own advocate when you can, have others to act for you when you can't. Be as physically active as you can. Like good sleep, exercise really speed up recovery.

• **NOTICE** the good and bad in your care, and speak up if you have any questions or concerns. Notice the little acts of kindness that make illness bearable, and be thankful for them.

• **GIVE BACK** to the NHS and your carers by providing thanks and constructive feedback. Share vital information with other patients and carers. Get involved in research, service improvement and design and volunteering for your local NHS and charities.

• **EAT WELL, RELAX, SLEEP** – These are even more important when you're ill. Take a face mask and good ear plugs into hospital. Sleep is often hardest when you need it most.

ABOUT THE AUTHOR
Dr Phil Hammond

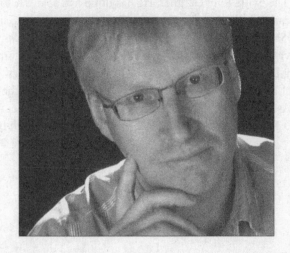

Phil Hammond is an NHS doctor, journalist, broadcaster, speaker, campaigner and comedian. He was a lecturer at the universities of Birmingham and Bristol, training medical students and doctors to communicate better with patients. This book draws on nearly thirty years of experience to do the reverse; help patients and carers cope better with life, illness and the NHS, and seek out the right care.

As a doctor, Phil has worked part time in general practice for over twenty years, and has also worked in sexual health. He currently works in a specialist NHS team for young people with chronic fatigue. Phil presented five series of *Trust Me, I'm a Doctor* on BBC2, encouraging patients to be more involved, assertive and questioning. He was a presenter for BBC Radio Bristol from 2006 to 2018, but was sacked when he announced that he might stand against Jacob Rees-Mogg at the next election. He is *Private Eye*'s medical correspondent, broke the story of the Bristol heart scandal in 1992 and gave evidence to the subsequent

Public Inquiry. In 2012, Phil was shortlisted, with Andrew Bousfield, for the Martha Gellhorn Prize for Journalism for 'Shoot the Messenger', a *Private Eye* investigation into the shocking treatment of NHS whistle-blowers.

As a comedian, Phil was half of the award-winning double-act Struck Off and Die, with Tony Gardner. He has done five solo UK tours and has appeared on *Have I Got News For You*, *Question Time*, *Countdown*, *The One Show* and *Long Live Britain*. His NHS comedy *Polyoaks*, written with David Spicer, has a fourth series on Radio 4. He is a columnist for the *Daily Telegraph*, and writes comment pieces for *The Times*. Phil is a patron of Meningitis UK, the Doctors' Support Network, the Herpes Viruses Association, Patients First, PoTS, the NET Patient Foundation, Kissing it Better and My Death, My Decision. This is his fifth book.

PREFACE

I've been fighting Crohn's disease for control of the body we both inhabit for as long as I can remember. I was finally diagnosed in the spring of 1983, when I was nineteen, after seeing seventeen different GPs in my desperate attempt to prove I wasn't a neurotic hypochondriac causing my own gut spasms, diarrhoea and blood loss. The relief of being told I had a 'real' disease cannot be overestimated. The fact that I was told I must have had it for fifteen years for it to be in the state it was, was air-punchingly satisfying. From then on, I have to say, my care from the NHS has been fantastic. Everything Nye Bevan could have hoped for. But I had to work to make that happen as well. You can't just sit back and hope the NHS will look after you; you have to stay on top of it.

Wendy Lee, writer

I'm very grateful for all the care I've received – the doctors and nurses have all been kind and mostly competent. But I just want to be free from the shackles of my illness and the NHS. I hate being dependent, I hate not being in control and I especially hate being at the mercy of a splintered, unreliable system that is organized around its own needs and not mine. The NHS and social care system needs some serious re-engineering.

Pat, seventy-six, retired engineer

All our science, measured against reality, is primitive and childlike – and yet it is the most precious thing we have.

Albert Einstein

There are lots of books written by doctors who have never been ill, telling people how to behave when they are. I hope I haven't fallen too deeply into this trap. I have managed to avoid a night in hospital (as a patient) in my fifty-three years, but I have experienced devastating loss (my Dad took his life when I was seven) and learned what it takes to recover and stay emotionally healthy. I've also learned that people cope with hardship and stressful situations in very different ways. Nobody can tell you how to think, feel or behave when you're ill or when you're caring for someone who's ill. But you can learn a lot from those who've been there.

Almost everyone hates being ill, hates the restrictions it places on their lives, the loss of control and the dependency on others. Illness can take up all your time, especially if you have to combine being ill with navigating the complexity and chaos of any healthcare system. The NHS is trying to shift the balance of power to patients, to give you more choice and control, but as healthcare gets more complex and high-tech, the power shifts back to those who control the technology. The internet is helping to democratize the NHS – to give you the information you need when you need it – but the choices about when, whether and how to treat are getting harder. Just because we can do something, doesn't mean we should. Everyone deserves a kind, gentle, humane death in the place of their choice but too many deaths are high-tech, inhumane and in hospital. The same applies to birth, but home birth is not without its risks too. The secret is to learn about and accept those risks, and – as always in the NHS – have a Plan B to cover any emergency.

Patients yearn to be free from illness and the NHS maze but so do many NHS staff. The mental and physical health of the workforce is poor, ironic for an organization that promotes health. Just as patients may fear pain, death and the limits that illness places on their lives, staff fear making a mistake, being blamed, and not being able to cope with demands and expectations. When errors occur, staff are sometimes fearful of telling the truth. And yet the NHS is built on trust, and you can't trust anyone who doesn't tell you the truth. Staff and patients need to feel free to be honest and open with each other, without fear of blame or judgement. We need to move from blind trust to kind truth.

Healthcare choices will always be complex and uncertain, science is always a simplification and what's right for one person, or what a doctor thinks is right for you, may not be what you think is right for you. Only you can decide how involved you want to be in decisions about your care, but some evidence suggests that the more involved you are, and are allowed to be, the more likely you are to get the right care for you. The overriding message of this book is that great health-care is all about kind, honest and trusting relationships, and they are two-way streets. You need to trust yourself to stay as healthy and as free as you can, live well with illness, seek help when you need to and try to share decisions in your treatment. And you need to develop good relationships with NHS staff who earn your trust and include you as central to a team focused on helping you live the life you want to.

There's much less published evidence of what patients can do to get better care if they aren't included as part of the team, or when trust, communication and respect break down and you're left to try to fix your own care in a splintered system that's creaking at the seams. It's possibly the hardest thing you'll ever have to do, particularly when you're weighed down with your own illness. But as the journalist Edward R Murrow observed: 'Difficulty is the excuse history never accepts.' We have to believe we can make our healthcare and health service even better and safer. Life without hope is horrid.

This book uses stories and advice patients and carers have shared with me, and also stories from *Patient Opinion*, *iWantGreatCare*, *healthtalk.org*, *PatientsLikeMe*, *Patients Know Best*, the NHS website, the charities I'm attached to and other health websites and blogs. It's not exposé, and it's about understanding not blame. Many patients are for-going their own right to confidentiality to share their diagnosis, story, tips and tactics with others – and to learn from them. When I qualified in 1987, patients often weren't shown the possible route maps for their care, and were certainly not allowed to touch the steering wheel. Now the internet is driving patient power, but you have to check it's taking you in the right direction.

We will each have to find our own way as a patient, if you haven't got there already, and nobody knows how you'll react when you get there – not even you. Bad news can lead to grief and any combination of shock, anger, numbness, denial or even laughter. But if you have reasons to stay alive (a person, a pet, a passion for peonies), the human spirit usually bounces back and tries to tackle illness and the NHS head on. Thank you to all those who have shared their stories to help and inspire others. Patients and carers are starting to lead the NHS in a bidet revolution, from the bottom up. This book is dedicated to you.

Phil Hammond
drphilhammond.com, @drphilhammond

NOTE: I am sure to have made errors in this book, and this may be its most important message. All humans make mistakes, more so when they're under pressure. The more you observe and get involved in your NHS care, the more human errors you will spot, correct and help us learn from. Your medical records are a great place to start. Mistakes are how we improve, but we can only do that if we're allowed to admit to error and talk it through without fear. Too often, a culture of blame in the NHS means mistakes are hidden and then repeated. Too often, patients are blamed for being ill, overweight or old rather than loved and helped to improve. Without kindness and honesty, healthcare is rotten.

1

The NHS and Us

- Healthy living is often more powerful at preventing illness than anything the NHS can offer.

- Ninety per cent of symptoms never reach the NHS.

- Ninety per cent of the symptoms that do reach the NHS are treated outside hospital.

- The average age of patients using NHS hospitals is over eighty, and in general practice it's seventy-five.

- All health services are facing the challenge of people living longer with illness.

- Demand for NHS services and social care is rising much faster than its current funding level. We need to pay more.

The **principle** of the NHS is both wonderful and simple. People should be cared for according to their needs, not their ability to pay. I would fight very hard to defend this.

The **purpose** of the NHS is also very simple. NHS care should improve your life and – when your time comes – improve your death. That doesn't have to be via high-tech treatment – often compassion, support, reassurance and the right information at the right time make a huge difference.

The **practicality** of the NHS and social care is that they are facing a multibillion pound black hole in their finances over the next decade, and beyond. If the economy picks up and we agree to put more money into it – then it may just about stay on the rails. But it's already struggling to cope with the demand, partly because it's a victim of its own success. Thanks to the NHS and improvements in public health and social care, we are living much longer with diseases that previously would have killed us.

I have no idea where the money will come from to safely fund NHS and social care in the future – and I doubt any politician does either, but we need to stop wasting precious resources. Waste is everyone's responsibility – patients, professionals and politicians – and a huge problem in the NHS. We waste vast sums on unnecessary reorganizations. Perhaps 20 per cent of mainstream clinical practice brings no benefit to patients and the cost of prescribed medicines wasted is around £300 million each year. And yet when patients are given time and support to understand the risks and benefits of tests and treatments, they usually choose less medicine not more. And when doctors aren't fearful of being blamed or sued, they use tests and treatments more wisely. We need to be more open about the costs and limits of healthcare, as well as its benefits.

The principle of the NHS must never change – it glues us together as a decent, humane society – so we need to focus on its purpose to get the best care possible from the limited resources available. And for an organization that spends over £120 billion of public money, we have surprisingly little evidence of how well it is spent. For most patients, we don't know whether NHS care made your life better, worse or no different. This information black hole is as big as the financial one.

Take a few minutes to consider your own, or your family's experience of the NHS. For each experience you can remember think:

- Did it benefit my life?

- How?

- Could the benefit have been greater?

- How?

- Could I have got the same benefit by using the NHS less, or not at all?

Benefits can come from friendship, compassion, reassurance, information and prevention – as well as treatment to help you, say, see or walk again. Unless you remind yourself – and the NHS – whether your healthcare improved your life, why and how, we have no way of improving the system or improving your care in the future. Prevention is trickier to judge. I'll never know if my blood pressure pills have prevented a stroke or heart attack, but they give me no side effects, my blood pressure has come down to normal and I feel more reassured taking them – which is as good as it gets for me..

Every modern industry spends a lot of money analysing its results and the NHS is trying to catch up. But to do so you have to tell us how your care was delivered and whether it made a difference to your life in the short term (e.g. 'I got out of hospital alive') and longer term (e.g. 'I am now able to get on the trampoline with my grandchildren'). So if you're asked to provide feedback about your care, please take the time to do it fairly and constructively (positive points first, suggestions for improvement after). The feedback I get from patients and carers motivates me to do the best job I can – and makes me proud to do that job – more than anything else. More importantly, honest feedback and the sharing of experiences helps patients and carers to prepare for what lies ahead, and to decide where and whether they want to be treated.

My own experiences of the NHS as a patient and carer have been overwhelmingly positive, and I've got into the habit of thanking the staff through feedback, and telling them which aspects of the care were most valuable. Usually, it's compassion, competence and good communication.

THE NHS IN PRACTICE

On any day, there are over a million consultations throughout the NHS – in homes and communities, general practice, hospital outpatients and wards, ambulances, emergency departments, sexual health clinics, dental surgeries, opticians and pharmacies and increasingly on the phone, online, by email, Skype and smartphone. Ten million decisions about patient care are made every day, often under intense time pressure and with imperfect information. Your best chance of getting the NHS care you need in these circumstances is to help make these decisions better, and to check if they're getting the desired results.

And you will need help too – people to help you navigate your way through what can be a complex and confusing system. This could be a friend, relative, nurse, GP, charity helpliner, another patient or yourself – or more likely a combination of people at different stages. A surprising number of tests and treatments don't have much effect on improving your life, so a savvy patient should always ask, 'How likely am I to benefit from this test or treatment?' and 'What is most likely to happen if we did nothing?' Often, the most likely answer is that you would live as long as you would have without it.

If you're lucky, take sensible risks and live a life of passion and purpose, you might reach eighty with barely a nod to the NHS. Or you may be unlucky and dependent on the NHS for long periods of your life. On one level, using the NHS is very simple. You want the right care for you, preferably first time, and if you're receiving care in lots of different places you want it all to join up and for the teams treating you to talk to each other. Just about everything goes through your GP, so if you haven't got one or can't easily get access to one, you're at a serious disadvantage. And if you've got one you know, like and trust who can sort most of your care out close to home, protect you from over-treatment but also point you in the direction of great NHS services when you need them, it's a huge advantage.

The NHS structure is so complex, confusing and ever changing – particularly in England – that most of the staff can't explain who's in charge and what all the organizations within it do. Many haven't even read the NHS Constitution, a clunky instruction manual for the NHS in England (although the principles apply throughout the UK). It only does half the job, because it tells you your rights and responsibilities without telling you how to get or fulfil them. It tells you what you should be getting, but sometimes it'll be up to you to fight very hard to get it. What I like about the Constitution is that it does not mention any political party. It's as if you've entered a dream world, based on values, principles and science, where all the tedious political infighting over the NHS had been surgically removed.

If we want an honest, humane and trustworthy NHS, it has to be informed by honest, humane and trustworthy politics. Politicians in all parties must grow up, collaborate and continuously improve the NHS based on scientific evidence and patient experience. To do that we must be honest about the harm it sometimes causes, and loudly praise the good it usually does. And we must be able to suck out the fear, and fix the harm openly and honestly without always having to blame someone for it.

In all four UK countries, there are large variations in the safety, quality and experiences of NHS and social care that you can help fix. There is evidence that informed, involved patients can get better care – although success is never guaranteed – and that by sharing your experiences, support and expertise, other patients can get better care too.

It's worth knowing your rights and responsibilities as set out in the NHS Constitution. If you've had excellent care in the NHS, it all makes perfect sense. If you've had poor care and felt powerless to put it right, it's much harder to stomach. Your rights, on close analysis, aren't quite as watertight as you might like.

Here's a summary.

Your Legal Rights in the NHS

- You have the right to access and receive NHS services free of charge.*

- You have the right not to be discriminated against.

- You have the right not to wait longer for treatment than agreed waiting times.*

- You have the right to be treated with a professional standard of care, by appropriately qualified and experienced staff, in a properly approved or registered organization that meets required levels of safety and quality.

* Terms and conditions apply. www.nhs.uk to read the Constitution in full.

- You have the right to drugs and treatments' that have been recommended by NICE for use in the NHS, if your doctor says they are clinically appropriate for you.**

- You have the right to receive approved vaccinations.

- You have the right to be treated with dignity and respect, in accordance with your human rights.

- You have the right to accept or refuse treatment that is offered to you, and not to be given any physical examination or treatment unless you have given valid consent.

- If you do not have the capacity to do so, consent must be obtained from a person legally able to act on your behalf, or the treatment must be in your best interests.***

- You have the right to be given information about the test and treatment options available to you, what they involve and their risks and benefits.

- You have the right of access to your own health records and to have any factual inaccuracies corrected.

- You have the right to privacy and confidentiality and to expect the NHS to keep your confidential information safe and secure.

- You have the right to be informed about how your information is used.

** NICE (the National Institute for Health and Care Excellence) is an independent organization producing guidance on drugs and treatments. 'Recommended for use by NICE' refers to a type of NICE recommendation set out in legislation. The NHS is obliged to fund specified NICE recommendations from a date no longer than three months from the publication of the recommendation unless, in certain limited circumstances, a longer period is specified.

*** If you are detained in hospital or on supervised community treatment under the Mental Health Act 1983 different rules may apply to treatment for your mental disorder. These rules will be explained to you at the time. They may mean that you can be given treatment for your mental disorder even though you do not consent.

- You have the right to request that your confidential information is not used beyond your own care and treatment and to have your objections considered, and where your wishes cannot be followed, to be told the reasons, including the legal basis.

- You have the right to choose your GP practice, and to be accepted by that practice unless there are reasonable grounds to refuse, in which case you will be informed of those reasons.

- You have the right to express a preference for using a particular doctor within your GP practice, and for the practice to try to comply.

- You have the right to make choices about the services commissioned by NHS bodies and to information to support these choices.*

- You have the right to be involved in discussions and decisions about your health and care, including your end of life care, and to be given information to enable you to do this. Where appropriate this right includes your family and carers.

- You have the right to be involved, directly or through representatives, in the planning of healthcare services commissioned by NHS bodies.*

- You have the right to have any complaint you make about NHS services acknowledged within three working days and to have it properly investigated.

- You have the right to discuss the manner in which the complaint is to be handled, and to know the period within which the investigation is likely to be completed and the response sent.

- You have the right to be kept informed of progress and to know the outcome of any investigation into your complaint, including an explanation of the conclusions and confirmation that any action needed in consequence of the complaint has been taken or is proposed to be taken.

- You have the right to take your complaint to the independent Parliamentary and Health Service Ombudsman or Local Government

* Terms and conditions apply. www.nhs.uk to read the Constitution in full.

Ombudsman, if you are not satisfied with the way your complaint has been dealt with by the NHS.

- You have the right to make a claim for judicial review if you think you have been directly affected by an unlawful act or decision of an NHS body or local authority.

- You have the right to compensation where you have been harmed by negligent treatment.

Along with your rights, the NHS Constitution outlines your responsibilities as an NHS patient. You could guess most of them – but do you do them?

Responsibilities of Patients and the Public Using the NHS

- Please recognize that you can make a significant contribution to your own, and your family's, good health and wellbeing, and take personal responsibility for it.

- Please register with a GP practice – the main point of access to NHS care as commissioned by NHS bodies.

- Please treat NHS staff and other patients with respect and recognise that violence, or the causing of nuisance or disturbance on NHS premises, could result in prosecution. You should recognise that abusive and violent behaviour could result in you being refused access to NHS services.

- Please provide accurate information about your health, condition and status.

- Please keep appointments, or cancel within reasonable time. Receiving treatment within the maximum waiting times may be compromised unless you do.

- Please follow the course of treatment which you have agreed, and talk to your clinician if you find this difficult.

- Please participate in important public health programmes such as vaccination.

- Please ensure that those closest to you are aware of your wishes about organ donation.

- Please give feedback – both positive and negative – about your experiences and the treatment and care you have received, including any adverse reactions you may have had. You can often provide feedback anonymously and giving feedback will not affect adversely your care or how you are treated. If a family member or someone you are a carer for is a patient and unable to provide feedback, you are encouraged to give feedback about their experiences on their behalf. Feedback will help to improve NHS services for all.

The NHS does not always deliver your rights, just as patients don't always live up to their responsibilities. But knowing what your rights are can give you the courage and confidence to speak up and to try to get your care back on track. And taking on as much responsibility as you can for your health and healthcare is your best chance of improving it.

THE PRESSURES FACED BY THE NHS

The good news is that every day, the vast majority of the 67 million people eligible to use the NHS, don't need to. And every day you don't need to use the NHS, someone else benefits. Most people are very capable of looking after themselves most of the time, self-treating for minor ailments and knowing when and where to seek help for serious illness. 90 per cent of symptoms are self-treated but an estimated fifty-two million visits to general practice each year are still for conditions that would get better with time. Self-care is likely to improve further when those who want it are given access to and control over their medical records and data, and technology is better used to direct you to the right information when you need it. In the meantime, a friendly pharmacist can often save you a trip to the GP.

The bad news is that demand in many areas outstrips both the supply of services and the funding for them. Patients who need care are having to wait longer for it, and too many referrals are rejected as not urgent enough, when the NHS should be doing its utmost to prevent emergencies. Here's an example from a consultant psychiatrist of the pressures facing his Child and Adolescent Mental Health Service:

'WE HAVE TO REFUSE OR DELAY MANY REFERRALS'

We get on average seventeen new referrals a day of young people with serious mental health issues. We are so overloaded and the staff are so stressed that many of them have gone off sick, making it even harder for those of us who remain. We simply have to refuse or delay many referrals even though I know young people need us and they will get worse without us. I may have to choose between seeing a young person who has self-harmed for a year, and a young person who has done it for a week. The person who has self-harmed for a year will be absolutely desperate, but I may be more likely to achieve a positive outcome for the person who has only harmed for a week. Who should I see? How do I allocate these precious NHS resources? Do we have to wait until a young person we've turned away commits suicide before somebody sits up and notices how we are struggling to cope? And we're struggling to cope because the communities our young people live in are struggling to cope. There is a very, very big mental illness iceberg out there and it's showing no signs of melting.

Life is tough enough for NHS staff, but imagine what it's like for these children and their carers who can't get any care at all? I speak to staff, patients and carers all over the UK, and the pattern of services struggling – or simply not being able to cope safely – with the demands placed on them is common across the NHS. Waiting times are creeping up, emergency departments are overflowing, people struggle to get a GP appointment, services are being restricted and rationed and lots of people are having to fend for themselves. This has been a recurring theme ever since I qualified as a doctor in 1987, and yet life expectancy for men and women has increased pretty much every year but since 2010 it has levelled off and the mortality rate for babies, children, the poor and the elderly has actually risen. We are not currently caring for our most vulnerable citizens as well as we should be.

The NHS is nearly always buckling under the demands placed on it, partly because it's a victim of its own success. Improvements in public health, wealth and healthcare since the NHS was founded sixty-seven years ago have been stunning. In 1948, half the population died before the age of sixty-five. Now, the average life expectancy is over eighty. One in three children born today will live to one hundred, but one in four boys born in Glasgow still won't make it to sixty-five. The UK is still a very unequal society, and the rich not only live fifteen years longer than the poor, but they have up to twenty years more healthy living. Life is very, very unfair, which is why we need to fight poverty and build the confidence, courage and resilience in our children to live well, as well as improve and fund the NHS. Those who pay for it most often use it least. It's the badge of honour for living in a humane society.

And we nearly all need it eventually if we want help or treatment. One in two people in the UK will get cancer, one in three will get diabetes and nearly everyone will get heart disease. Many of these diseases will be contained rather than cured. Obesity appears unstoppable. Liver disease, kidney disease, lung disease, musculoskeletal disease, depression and anxiety are all on the increase. Mental illnesses cost the UK over £70 billion a year, one in three of us experiences mental health problems every year and one in three people over sixty-five will die with dementia. Many people with dementia live for many years, even if they haven't been diagnosed and treated. Dementia alone already costs the economy more than cancer and heart disease put together.

These chronic diseases account for 70 per cent of the NHS budget, although many can be delayed if not prevented by a healthier lifestyle. Those with three or more incurable diseases are usually on multiple medications, the combined effects of which are unknown. Many older patients on multiple drugs struggle to take them properly, and there's a delicate balance between benefit and harm. Loneliness is often a far bigger problem.

The NHS and social care system is crucially dependent on millions of unpaid volunteers and carers, and many very dedicated but poorly paid care workers. The round-the-clock pressures and responsibilities they face are huge. If carers went on strike, the NHS and social care service would collapse overnight. Keeping it all afloat is a massive, collaborative effort and we are far too reliant on institutionalized care, rather than supporting people in their homes.

More women give birth in hospital than need or want to be there, so those who really need to have hospital births don't always get safe care. Far too many frail elderly patients, many with dementia, end up in acute hospitals, often the most frightening and disorientating place they can be. Far too many people with mental illness end up in police custody and far too many people die in hospital when they want to die at home. We can change this, if services join up, and patients and carers receive the right training and support. Having chemotherapy or dialysis at home can transform not just your healthcare but your whole life. It doesn't happen nearly enough.

Fixing the NHS and social care system will not be quick or easy, even if we put more money in. In many instances, it would often be kinder to have less high-tech, expensive intervention than more. Despite the obvious pressures the NHS is under, I remain optimistic about its future because I meet so many brilliant, innovative, dedicated people working in it, and so many inspirational and supportive people using it, many of whom want to do more for themselves if they were allowed. If all we ever did in the NHS was capture the ideas and feedback from frontline staff, patients and carers, and use it to continuously improve a stable system that everyone understood, the NHS would be out of sight as the world's best. We have to spend every available penny supporting and joining up the frontline – the NHS is not about the bricks and mortar, it's about mobilizing and motivating a brilliant workforce to serve patients and give you as much control as you want over your care. And to do that, you need to find your voice and we need to listen to you.

Research done by the Health Foundation, *When Doctors and Patients Talk*, found that NHS staff are often as anxious and fearful as you are during consultations. They are anxious and frightened of missing an important diagnosis, not being able to give patients what they are entitled to, not being able to practise the standards of care they'd like to, having to deal with justifiable anger, missing a target they have been ordered to hit, being asked to do something they do not feel competent to do, or having to look after so many patients in such a short space of time they just do not feel safe. The ever-present fear is that they simply cannot cope safely with the demand. Just as we shouldn't blame people for being ill or old or overweight, we shouldn't blame NHS staff for not being able to always provide the highest standards of care. Praise, kindness and understanding are much better motivators.

To improve, the NHS needs to be simplified so that anyone can understand it. We pretend to distinguish between healthcare and social care, but it's all 'care' and it should be joined into one care system, with those with the greatest need treated by one team with one named person responsible for coordinating your care. And we must all do everything we can to live well. In the NHS, the staff spend too much time diving into the river of illness, pulling people out and trying to put them back together that no-one has time to wander upstream and look at who's pushing you in.

2

Staying Alive

LIVING WITH RELISH

Tell me, what is it you plan to do with your one wild and precious life?
Mary Oliver

Precious time is slipping away, and our lives are over in the blink of a geological nanosecond. No-one ever said on their deathbed, they wish they'd spent more time finding their way around the NHS. What you can do for yourself to live well is often far greater than anything medical science or the NHS can do for you, and taking the knowledge, skills, passion and courage you've learned in life into the NHS gives you the best chance of thriving and surviving when you need to use it.

Do CLANGERS every day

Connect
Learn
(BE) **A**ctive
Notice
Give back
Eat well
Relax
Sleep

In 2008, research by the New Economics Foundation and funded by the government, came up with five evidence-based steps we can all take to improve our mental wellbeing. Connect, Learn, be Active, Notice and Give back (CLANG). I built on this to come up with a plan for 'whole-body wellbeing' by adding Eat well, Relax and Sleep. These are the fundamentals of feeling good, and, if you can do them at regular times to fit in with your body's natural 24 hour rhythm (particularly eating, exercising and sleeping), it will do more to improve your health and aid your recovery than any drug I could prescribe. Above all, CLANGERS are fun and joyful to do. And the very act of doing them makes you healthier.

• **CONNECT** with the world around you. Human beings are social animals. We are leaves on a tree, needing to feel part of something bigger. Reach out to people, pets, plants, places and the planet. These connections are the cornerstones of our life. Take time and care to nurture them. Disconnection and loneliness may be as bad for us as smoking. I recently got all my audience members to hug the people either side of them. A man came up to me after the show and thanked me. 'That's the only hug I've had all year.' There may be people living near you who go for months without any human touch. And don't forget to connect with yourself. Loving yourself may not always be easy, but are you happy in your skin? Can you enjoy your own company? Can you disappear inside your own head and not mind what you find there? Can you get through a night on your own without two bottles of wine and Netflix? People who like their own company like being on their own sometimes. Loneliness becomes solitude. You have space to think, reflect, explore and relax.

• **LEARN** What do you want to do with your one wild and precious life? A purpose in life often stems from learning about what matters most to you, developing a passion for learning and keeping your curiosity alive. And there is good evidence that the more you learn, the better your health becomes. Try something new. Rediscover an old interest. Sign up for that course. Join a choir. Take on a different responsibility at work. Fix a bike. Learn to play an instrument or how to cook your favourite food. Set a challenge you will enjoy achieving. Learning new things will make you more confident as well as being fun. And learning with others in your 'circle' often cements the skills and gives you confidence to use your new knowledge. Curious people always have a reason to get out of bed. When you're ill, transfer these learning skills to the NHS. Keep that curiosity going. Ask to see your cancer under a microscope. The fear may melt away in a sea of purple.

• **BE ACTIVE** in mind and body. Rediscover activities and passions you left behind, and have the courage to try new ones. Aim for five portions of fun a day, each different, at least one outdoors and one that involved getting pleasantly breathless. Being outdoors in the morning light wakes you up and helps you sleep well later. Gardening, dancing or singing in a choir are all excellent therapy. Physical activity is better for both mind and body than any drug, but keeps you awake if you do it within 2 hours of bed time. Choose activities that you enjoy, so you want to keep doing them. Park runs, dancing, singing, cycling and gardening are great examples. And let's not forget the power of pets. For most symptoms, you may be better off with a dog than a doctor. Dogs are always happy to see you. Dogs give you unconditional love. If you hug a dog it reduces your blood pressure. They can also reduce your cholesterol (by eating your food). Dogs look you in the eye (not even your husband does that) and they keep looking at you until you take them out for a walk. You get exercise, the beautiful outdoors and friendship from other dog owners. And you can wrestle on the carpet with a dog without getting arrested. When did you have that much fun with a doctor?

• **NOTICE** and be present in, the world around you. Fill up your senses. Catch sight of the beautiful. Remark on the unusual. Enjoy the everyday. Savour the moment, and your place in it. Life is a balance and being and doing, and the older and wiser we get, we realise that most of the pleasure in life comes from just being. Notice how lovely your partner or children are without judging or diagnosing them. Simply slowing down and focusing on your breathing for ten minutes a day can pay huge dividends. Breathe in for 3, hold for 4 and out for 5. Feel those fabulous human air bags filling up to their fullest extent. Then slowly, slowly let it all out.

• **GIVE BACK** Helping and caring for friends, strangers and those less fortunate than ourselves is fundamental to good emotional health. It cements us as part of a community and develops more meaningful connections and insights. A friend of mine overheard a dad telling a waiter in the Glasgow hotel that is son was having chemotherapy in the nearby hospital, and that he was going to shave his head in solidarity so they would both be bald when they came down to breakfast in the morning. He wanted to warn the waiters so they didn't feel uncomfortable. The head waiter said he would pass the message on. When the newly bald father walked into the restaurant with his son the following morning, they looked around and saw that every single waiter had shaved his head. The joy of being human is to be humane.

• **EAT WELL** Food is above all a pleasure. Learn what's good and enjoyable to eat, and in what quantities. Learn how to grow it, where to buy it and how to prepare it. Set time aside to sit and eat with friends and family. Your gut is like a garden. It contains trillions of healthy bacteria that are as fundamental to your health as your DNA. Many people with chronic diseases have a fairly narrow range of bacteria in the gut. Healthier people seem to have a wider range of bacteria fed from a wide variety of different foods. Eat plenty of plants – vegetables and fruits of many different types and colours, nuts, seeds, whole grains and olive oil. Add in a little bit of what you fancy. Sustainable fish, lean meat, dark chocolate and the odd beer or glass of wine (note: alcohol can improve your chat but seriously disrupt your sleep). You can have the odd Pringle but you wouldn't plant too many in your garden. Cutting down on sugary snacks and drinks, processed food is a good starting point. Learn to love water as your 'go to' drink. And try to do all your eating in a 12 hour period (say 7am-7pm) to fit in with your body clock, give your gut a break and improve your sleep

• **RELAX** Take time to rest and reflect on the day you've had, reliving and re-savouring the happy memories and having gratitude for friends and family. Learn to meditate. Be kind to your mind and let it wind down and de-clutter. My Uncle Ron used to have a sitting room that was just for sitting. At the end of the day, he would recall happy little things that have happened during the day, and be grateful for the love he had in his life. I used to think he was crazy, but I now know he was practising positive psychology. Our brains are neuro-plastic, which means what we focus on is what grows. So if we learn to relive happy moments and have gratitude for the good things, it can actually make us happier. And this happy end of day wind down can really improve your sleep.

• **SLEEP** Good sleep is one of life's great joys. It's also essential for mental and physical health, helping you prevent and recover from a whole range of illnesses and improving your energy levels, creativity and performance. The flip side is that sleep deprivation kills both in the short term (e.g. driving or doctoring while sleep deprived) and in the longer term (the less you sleep, the shorter your life expectancy). If the doctor or nurse treating you is sleep deprived, then the risk they will make a mistake in your care is considerably higher. Adults work best on a regular 8 hours sleep a night, adolescents and children need more. If you need to be convinced about the need for good sleep, read *Why We Sleep* by Matthew Walker. Below are the tips I give to my patients.

24 WAYS TO TRY TO IMPROVE YOUR SLEEP

1. Try to go to bed at the same time and wake up at the same time each day, including weekends, aiming for 8 hours sleep every night. This is important but not easy, so decide which timing works best for you and your daily functioning. You will need to protect 8.5 hours to give you adequate nodding off time.

2. If this goes wrong, don't beat yourself up. If you don't get good, refreshing sleep you will build up a sleep debt that has to be paid off on days off.

3. If you are asleep all day and awake at night, treat this like jetlag and cut back your going to bed time and your waking up time by 1 hour each day. Day One: sleep at 6 am, wake at 3 pm. Day Two: sleep at 5 am, wake at 2 pm. Day Three: sleep at 4am, wake at 1 pm, and so on until you wake at the desired time.

4. Have the right sunlight exposure. Daylight is key to regulating daily sleep patterns. Try to get outside in natural sunlight for at least thirty minutes each day. If you aren't sensitive to light wake up with the sun or use bright lights in the morning. Sleep experts recommend that, if

you have problems falling asleep, you should get an hour of exposure to morning sunlight and turn down the lights before bedtime.

5. Enforce a strict 'no caffeine after noon' rule. Coffee, colas, certain
   teas, and chocolate contain the stimulant caffeine, and its effects
   can take as long as twelve hours to wear off fully. Nicotine in cigarettes and e-cigarettes, and alcohol also severely disrupts your sleep,
   as can some medications. Check with your pharmacist.

6. Come off close-up screens and games 60-90 minutes before bed.
   The blue light and excitement they give off boosts cortisol and
   blocks melatonin release.

7. Set an alarm to tell you when it's time for bed, and stick to it. Alarm
   clocks in the morning freak out your heart and are best avoided if
   possible.

8. Fit blackout blinds in your bedroom. The darker your room for sleep,
   the better. A black-out mask is a cheaper option.

9. Remove ALL screens from your bedroom, so temptation is avoided.

10. Consider opening the bedroom window. The perfect temperature for
    sleeping is around 17°C/65°F. A cooler room is much better for sleep-
    ing than a hot one

11. Eat earlier in the day, before 7 pm if possible. Don't snack at night.

12. Exercise earlier in the day, and outdoors when you can. Exercising 2
    hours before sleep time raises your metabolic rate and temperature,
    and makes it hard to sleep

13. Socializing is important but don't do it late at night except on special
    occasions.

14. Buy red lights for night-time illumination.

15. Buy amber glasses to filter blue light from screens.

16. Don't use your phone as an alarm clock.

17. Install f:lux on your e-devices, or switch on 'night-time mode' from 6pm.

18. Don't take catnaps after 3 pm and keep them short (no more than an hour).

19. Relax before bed. Don't overschedule your evening so that no time is left for unwinding. A relaxing activity, such as reading, listening to music, chatting through the day with friends or family or stroking a pet should be part of your bedtime ritual.

20. Take a hot bath before bed. The drop in body temperature after getting out of the bath may help you feel sleepy, and the bath can help you relax and slow down so you're more ready to sleep.

21. If you can't sleep, counting sheep isn't as effective as repeating the same word over and over (the, the, the, the...) or filling your mind with peaceful music (I listen to Sleep by Max Richter).

22. Don't lie in bed awake. If you find yourself still awake after staying in bed for more than twenty minutes or if you are starting to feel anxious or worried, get up and do some relaxing activity until you feel sleepy. The anxiety of not being able to sleep can make it harder to fall asleep.

23. Keep trying to improve your sleep, little by little. Sleeping pills are not the answer.

24. We all have bad runs of sleep, particularly in stressful times, but if we allow ourselves to get back in synch with our body clock, we can rediscover the joy of a good night's sleep.

LIVING WITH RISK

We all live with risk every day, but we deal with it in very different ways.

1. If you live in the UK, or indeed any country that disposes of its sewage properly, there's a good chance you'll live to eighty even if you go nowhere near the NHS. A lot of men, and a surprising number of doctors, adopt that approach. They run free, and keep on running until something bad happens.

2. If you do CLANGERS every day, you'll increase your chances of emotional health and a satisfied mind, and lower your risk of anxiety and the misery of comparing yourself with others rather than enjoying their company. Love and be loved.

3. If you want to improve your odds further, don't smoke, go easy on sugar and alcohol, love your fruit and veg, get breathless most days and try to keep your waist circumference (measured at the level of your tummy button, not your hips) at half your height or less. You're not only more likely to make it to eighty, but far more likely to live most of those years in good health rather than restricted by illness or trying to find an NHS parking space.

Many of the people I know who do this live great lives with barely a nod to the NHS. They're not all wealthy, but are genetically lucky, have enough money to live on, are free from fear and persecution, have learned to sort out their own symptoms and have the resilience and support to rebound from misfortune. Above all, they know that what they can do for themselves to stay healthy is usually far more powerful and enjoyable than anything the NHS can do for them. And they know that life is much richer being a groovy man or woman than a grumpy one.

You can live a great life without dwelling too long on your risks of early death and disease, or you may want to give them more thought. The current UK life expectancy of around eighty is an average, and roughly half of us will live longer and half of us will have shorter lives. The same applies for the number of years of good health you have. The healthiest people in the UK have twenty more years lived in good health than the least healthy. It's a truly shocking statistic. A lot of this is down to wealth, genetic make-up and good luck, but we can all raise our own personal bar, little by little, to live longer in good health. To do this, you need to consider what's most likely to harm your health. It's important to get risks in perspective, so you don't reach for a cigarette because you're worried by the headlines about a mutant virus in an Albanian ostrich abattoir.

Turn the page to see the risks leading to death in the UK in order of size. The larger the lettering, the larger the risk.

Smoking
High Blood Pressure
High Cholesterol
Obesity and Sugar
Low Fruit and Vegetables
Physical Inactivity
Alcohol
Suicide Risks (Poverty, Isolation, Stress, Abuse)
Non-transport Accidents
Infections
Transport Accidents

Pollution

Illicit Drug Use

Murder

Pregnancy and Birth

Medical Complications

War

These death risks are in average order for the whole UK population. The order in your personal risk league table will depend on your work, lifestyle and circumstances, and your risk of early death or disease is also strongly dependent on your age, sex and genes, which at present we can't do much about. You can pay privately to have your DNA examined for a 'best guess' report on your future disease risks, but that may just make you ill with anxiety. Some genetic risks are so strongly inherited that illness is inevitable. Whether and when you want to know in advance requires some careful thought.

The same applies to health checks and screening – there's a payoff between trying to pick up risks or diseases at an early stage to stop them worsening, and over-treating and scaring you for minimal or no benefit. The beauty of lifestyle and behaviour changes is that you can do many of them yourself, a little at a time, without turning you into a patient, and they're often far more fun and effective than medical screening and treatment. Just don't blame or beat yourself up if you don't always succeed. Failure is how we learn and improve, in and out of the NHS.

Time is precious, so if you want to cut your risks, focus on the big ones, not on whatever happens to be in the headlines today. You know if you smoke, and it's the biggest risk in the UK for early disease and death. If you can stop smoking for twenty-eight days, you are five times more likely to stay smoke-free for good, and if you can't do it alone the NHS can help you. It's one of the best, most effective and underrated services it offers: www.nhs.uk/smokefree.

Many people who take big risks with their health feel socially excluded and struggle to get help. If that's you, then a great charity may be better at helping you to turn your life around than the NHS (although you'll often need help from both). I've met people whose lives have been transformed with the support of charities such as Alcoholics Anonymous and Overeaters Anonymous. I've done work for a wonderful charity called Developing Health and Independence which helps people who are socially excluded for reasons such as homelessness, alcohol or drug problems, learning disabilities or emotional difficulties – and supports them to live well and help others. They succeed by tackling both the causes and consequences of social exclusion through practical and emotional support. They offer information, advice, supported housing away from the wrong crowd, counselling from professionals and those who've kicked their bad habits, social activities and work and training opportunities. The NHS could learn a huge amount from charities on how to join up services and support people to improve their lives, rather than just treat their illnesses. There are lots of other ways that aren't too much hassle, both to reduce your risk of harm and to improve your life. You can start by being wise to the risks of fire, water, falls, traffic, germs, tooth decay, sex, infectious disease and chronic disease. And then do easy things to reduce your risks (e.g. seatbelts, smoke alarms, stair-gates, vaccinations, condoms, tooth-brushing, hand-washing, food preparation, teaching your kids to cook, swim and learn life support, learning the red flag symptoms for cancer, heart disease, stroke, diabetes, dementia and mental illness). Life without any risk would be very dull, but serious injury or illness caused by an easily preventable risk is a tragedy. Many accidents and illnesses are preventable, and the sooner you spot a medical emergency and seek help, the better your chances of recovery.

Finally, and most importantly, be wise to the people around you. Talk to people in your workplace and community, but remember also to listen. Talk to someone if you're feeling distressed or upset. Help a friend or neighbour. If you or someone you know is at risk of taking their life, get urgent help. People who say they are going to kill themselves will often try, and too often succeed. It's very important to remember that people do not have to be, or appear, deeply depressed to commit suicide. The NHS isn't always quick enough to respond, but Samaritans are always there, twenty-four hours a day (08457 90 90 90, jo@samaritans.org). The risks of kindness even to strangers are tiny, but the benefits of just being there can be huge.

Using Medicine to Reduce Your Risks

If you remain mentally and physically active throughout your life and do CLANGERS every day, you'll live with relish and reduce your risks of disease and death without many tests or treatments. If you spot a miracle cure or death scare in the newspaper and want to find out more, the NHS has a great 'Behind the Headlines' webpage that will cut through the spin and bias and give you the bottom line. Charities such as Cancer Research UK and Macmillan are also excellent sources of information for the truth behind cancer scares and cures.

For example, in August 2014, a lot of newspapers suggested taking a daily aspirin to reduce your risk of cancer. It's a cheap-as-chips drug that's been around for years, comes from willow bark and on the face of it is a very simple way of reducing your risk of something very unpleasant. The headlines were universally positive:

- Daily aspirin 'cuts bowel and stomach cancer deaths' (BBC News).

- Taking Aspirin daily significantly reduces risk of cancer new study finds (*Mirror*).

- Aspirin should be taken by all over fifties to cut thousands of cancer deaths: study (*The Daily Telegraph*).

- Miracle pill aspirin could even ward off major cancers: Long-term use of the drug can cut chance of developing disease by up to a third (*Mail Online*).

- Daily dose of aspirin 'can cut the risk of cancer', says study (*The Independent*).

However, the statistical summary according to CRUK's website is far more realistic . . .

Aspirin can save lives, but there is a risk. If 1,000 people aged sixty take aspirin every day for ten years:

- Up to seventeen lives would be saved by preventing cancers and heart attacks

- Two to three deaths would be caused by strokes and bleeding

- 980 would live as long as they would have done without taking aspirin

We don't yet know:

- The dose to take

- How long to take it

- How to identify who shouldn't take it

So by far the most likely outcome if you take a daily aspirin is that you will live as long as you would have done without taking it, but if you had a family history of one of the cancers, or if you have heart disease, the benefits are likely to be greater. I'm not in those groups, so I don't take it (yet) – but I might if more studies come along to give me more bits of the jigsaw.

In truth, for many prescription drugs, a lot of patients taking them live just as long as if they didn't take them. If you're good with numbers and being offered a test or treatment, always ask, 'How likely am I to benefit from this?' and 'What is most likely to happen if we did nothing?' Then you can decide whether you think it's right for you or whether you'll take the risk of living without medicalization.

Reducing Risks Through Screening

Screening and health checks, like many medical interventions, aren't quite as effective as you've been led to believe but they can sometimes be life-savers. The aim is to catch a serious disease at an early stage when it can be treated to stop harm. But in doing so, we cause some harm to many more patients who have treatment that does not give them any benefit at all. And although we could probably prevent lots of diseases (at a cost) if everyone had screening that was known to be effective, your individual odds (the number of people like you who need to have screening to prevent one nasty disease) are often high.

The NHS decides what screening programmes and health checks it will offer, often based in imperfect science. And you have to decide whether you want them. A major problem with our existing screening programmes is that they were introduced in a culture of paternalism, where doctors or the Department of Health knew best and told women that they 'should' come forward for screening. Indeed, we were so one-sidedly positive about breast and cervical screening that we neglected to mention that – even in the best hands – it could never pick up every problem or prevent every case of cancer, and given the pressures those in the NHS work under, there would always be some human error in the interpretation of the results. It's only recently, when various scandals have dented our faith in doctors and the NHS, that you are seeing the downside of screening. There will always be many more 'abnormal smears' than cases of cervical cancer, and yet many women worry about even small changes. And there is always a risk that women will receive treatment for 'early changes' that would never have progressed to cancer if left alone.

As with most medicine, it's all about managing risk and uncertainty and – more importantly – how doctors and patients communicate. I don't tell women they 'should' have screening, but I point out the pros and cons and let them make a decision. If you choose not to have screening, there is still plenty you can do to reduce your risk of getting cancer or heart disease, such as stopping smoking, being active every day and keeping your weight and alcohol consumption in check. However, if screening programmes are to be worthwhile, they have to be properly funded and that includes putting aside time to explain to patients about the uncertainties as well as the potential benefits. It's your choice and you can make the decision alone, share it with others or do what your doctor or nurse recommends.

Whatever the screening programme you're invited to, ask about the balance of benefit and risk. You could ask about the (average) 'number needed to screen' to prevent one case of disease, and the (average) 'number needed to harm' to cause one unnecessary side effect, then weigh up the odds.

Breast Cancer Screening
Let's look at 1,000 women over a twenty-year period:

- If these women were not screened for breast cancer, fifty-eight out of 1,000 would be diagnosed with the disease.

- Of these fifty-eight women, twenty-one would die from breast cancer, thirty-seven would be treated and survive their disease. Seventeen would live healthy lives not affected by their cancer.

- If these women were screened for breast cancer, seventy-five out of 1,000 would be diagnosed with the disease.

- Of these seventy-five women, sixteen would die from breast cancer and fifty-nine would be treated and survive their disease. Five lives

would be saved by screening and seventeen would be over-diag-
nosed due to screening. That means they would be treated for breast
cancers that are real, but that would not have caused them any harm.

- So, for every life that is saved by breast cancer screening, three
  women are treated who didn't need to be. Each year, that means
  1,300 lives are saved in the UK but 4,000 women are treated when
  there would've been no harm.

- By far the most likely result if you choose breast screening is that it
  will be normal. However, a few very unlucky women will die from
  breast cancer despite screening.

Cervical Cancer Screening

There has never been a randomized controlled trial of cervical cancer
screening – the gold standard test to see if something works – so we
can't be absolutely sure of the figures. At a best guess, if you screen
10,000 women over twenty years for cervical cancer, you save ten
lives. Of those 10,000 women, 1,000 get letters telling them that they
have abnormalities and need repeat tests, more than 500 require col-
poscopies and biopsies with a small risk this may lead to premature
labour in later pregnancies. However, screening will also pick up and
treat some unpleasant cancers before they cause more damage. But it
can cause a lot of anxiety and you have to accept that risk as the price
you pay for a small reduction in your risk of a nasty cancer. Cervical
cancer is caused by the HPV virus – passed on during sex – and its risk
is greatly increased by smoking. So stopping smoking and using condoms are good ways to cut your risk, and the HPV vaccination
programme should too (although treatments never work quite as brilliantly in the long term as advertised).

Prostate Cancer Screening

This doesn't yet exist in the NHS, even though the disease kills 11,000
men a year. Less than 1,000 women die from cervical cancer each year,
so it seems illogical. Screening standards have tightened up over time
and if we started today, we might not introduce cervical cancer screening either.

The trouble with prostate cancer is that the behaviour of the cancer is difficult to predict. In some it spreads rapidly and presents too late for a cure, but in many others it remains localized in the prostate gland without causing any obvious harm. For the latter, surgery or radiotherapy may do more harm than good, because of the risk of causing incontinence or impotence. And the screening tests we have at present can't distinguish between the harmless ('pussy cat') cancers and the aggressive ('tiger') cancers.

A recent European study found that prostate screening could save 2,300 lives a year in the UK, but twenty-seven men would have to undergo treatment for each life saved, leaving thousands needlessly suffering distressing side effects. This is why we don't have a national screening programme – the committee that looks at the evidence decided that the harm from screening would outweigh the benefits (www.screening.nhs.uk/prostatecancer).

The race is on to develop better screening tests that identify those early cancers that are more likely to spread. In the meantime, it's left to men to decide for themselves whether they want to be assessed for prostate cancer or not. Black men are at higher risk as are those with a family history of the disease and it's certainly worth speaking to your GP about the pros and cons of PSA (prostate specific antigen) screening for you. For men above the age of fifty, there's a risk management programme you can check to decide whether to ask for the test or not (www.cancerscreening.nhs.uk/prostate/index.html).

If you ask different specialists, you get different answers. Some say all men over fifty should ask for a PSA test because even though it isn't perfect, the change in your PSA over time is a good way of tracking your risk of cancer, so having a baseline level done is worthwhile. Others say that PSA stands for Promoting Stress and Anxiety, and should be left well alone unless you are at increased risk of the disease.

Ultimately, it depends on how good you are at living with uncertainty. As technology advances, both the diagnosis and the treatment of prostate cancer gets better, with lots of options now available ranging from active surveillance and MRI scanning to localized radioactive seeds and robot-assisted surgery with fewer side effects. All of these options carry their own uncertainties, and the maths isn't simple. But then we're used to making complex choices in our life all the time, and we need to step up to the plate in the consulting room and have a grown-up conversation about what medicine can and can't do for us, rather than just fall back on 'what would you do doctor?' If you feel fine and live well, you could avoid all screening – and the anxiety it brings – if you can live with the slightly increased risk of having a silent killer. Or you can weigh up the pros and cons, climb aboard the screening rollercoaster and see where it takes you. You decide. (I'm fifty-three and my PSA is normal.)

Bowel Cancer Screening

I will be having this when my time comes (in three years). It simply involves taking a tiny sample of your poo and sending it off to be checked for blood that can't be seen. About 98 per cent of people will receive a normal result, and will be invited for screening again two years later. If your result is abnormal, you'll be invited to have further tests. This will usually involve a colonoscopy (flexible telescope up the bottom), which isn't huge fun but is done under sedation, takes less than half an hour and you'll be able to go home within a couple of hours. Even if you do have an abnormal first screening test, it doesn't necessarily mean you have cancer. Bleeding can be due to other causes, and many people who go on to have further tests will be relieved to find they don't have cancer after all.

Everyone aged sixty to sixty-nine in England, Wales and parts of Northern Ireland (fifty to seventy-four in Scotland – the cancer is more common there) is invited to take part every two years. If you're over seventy, you can still be screened if you call 0800 7076060 and ask for a testing kit. The reason I'll have this one is that bowel cancer is common – 36,000 cases a year in the UK and 18,000 deaths – and screening has been shown to improve survival rates by 16 per cent (by picking up the cancer before it spreads). Four out of five people who get colon cancer are over sixty, which is why the screening is aimed at them. If I needed a colonoscopy, however, I'd check that the person doing it had done lots of them and could prove he or she was competent – or was being trained by someone who was.

LIVING WITH RUST

We are all rusting to death, but we can slow it down.

> People talk about the temptations and dangers of 'fast food' but you can't get much faster than a banana. Okay, you have to peel it. Wash an apple and off you go. It's cheaper than a Mars bar. Raw broccoli. Carrots. All a lot faster than standing in a queue for processed gunk.

> I have a fridge magnet that says – 'if in doubt don't put it in your mouth'. It makes me laugh and pause to consider if I'm hungry or just moody. And it works in other social situations too (although we don't have much sex in the kitchen these days).

> Any cake that isn't freshly baked is chemical cake. Chemical cake sounds disgusting, tastes disgusting and it is disgusting. I still eat it, occasionally, but much less than I used to since I started calling it chemical cake.

> I've got this theory about taste buds. I think they regenerate every few months so if you wean yourself off, say, sweet tastes for a few months, your taste buds and brain adapt, and you don't miss sweet at all. Works for me.

> If you want to know what a portion size should be, turn your plate over and eat off the base.

> Walking is the most powerful mind and body drug ever invented, and with the fewest side effects. They should put it in the water.

> If you're a bloke and you can't see your penis, it's time to get a grip.

Although we have one of the best health services, at least in the Commonwealth Fund survey, the UK scored next to bottom on healthy living. Only America is an unhealthier, and more unequal, place to live than the United Kingdom. The NHS will continue to struggle unless we do more to eradicate poverty. The poorer you are the more likely you are to live a long time with illness, yet die before your time. But whatever level you're starting at, you can raise the bar on your health, little by little. Small changes in time add up to big changes. And every day you live well and don't need to use the NHS, somebody else benefits. It's the ultimate win-win.

I was introduced to the idea that we're all rusting to death by Michael Mosley, who I worked with on BBC2's *Trust Me, I'm A Doctor*. There is a fair bit of truth behind the theory outlined below. Michael has co-written two excellent books, *Fast Diet* and *Fast Exercise*, which are ideal for people who like to know the evidence behind how they should eat and exercise, as well as practical plans that can fit in with even the most chaotic lives. I can't better Michael's advice but I would add that you may have to tackle the mind rust before you can move on to the body rust. You need a passion for life and a motive to live well.

But think how far we've come in two billion years. Back then, there was the worst outbreak of pollution earth has ever known. Bacteria learnt how to use sunlight to convert water into food. This chemical process produced an extremely toxic gas as a by-product, which was intensely corrosive and destroyed most living things as it was released into the atmosphere. Over tens of millions of years the levels of this poison built up and up, from virtually nothing to almost 21 per cent of the entire atmosphere. That gas is oxygen, formed as bacteria split water and combined hydrogen with carbon to form simple sugars for food. They had no use for the oxygen, so they just let it go. Plant life later evolved to use this trick of photosynthesis.

For animals, oxygen is essential for life, but it's still very toxic. It reacts hungrily with proteins and enzymes, stopping them from working. It burns and destroys. If the levels of oxygen in our atmosphere rose much above current levels, we'd all die very young. The reason this doesn't happen is because other bacteria developed an even smarter chemical trick. They learnt how to convert oxygen, the great poison, into energy. Animals have inherited that evolutionary trick from them. But it's a Faustian pact. Oxygen keeps us alive, but it also destroys living tissue. The damage oxygen does to cells is the main reason why we age. It slowly rusts us to death. And the less care we take of ourselves, the quicker we rust.

When we use oxygen to produce energy, this process generates a group of particularly vicious chemicals called free radicals. Once

generated these free radicals and other oxidants, such as hydrogen per-
oxide, surge around your body. They damage arteries, which leads first
to the formation of fatty deposits, then narrowing of the arteries, then
heart attacks. It's that initial damage that starts everything else; if it
wasn't for free radicals it wouldn't really matter what your cholesterol
levels were, normal fat does not get deposited in healthy arteries. These
oxidants also get into your cells and damage your DNA. If your body
fails to repair this DNA damage then the cell may become abnormal,
and may turn into a cancer. Smoking increases the level of circulating
oxidants, and that's one way it causes heart disease and cancer.

We have in-built natural antioxidants in the form of enzymes which
help suppress the build-up of free radicals and there is some evidence
that people who have naturally high levels of antioxidants live longer
and have less disease. Your best chance of slowing down the rust is a
healthy diet and an active life, but you've got to figure out a way that
works for you. Once you do, the benefits can be huge. For great advice
and support, check out Change4Life on the NHS website.

I WANT TO BE FREE

When I grow old I want to be free-range elderly not battery elderly.
My mum used to take hens from the local battery farm, and we let
them just run free in the garden. It always amazed me how little time
it took for them to go from being dazed, depressed and confused to
getting a life and some feathers. I guess it's a bit like being freed after
a long period of torture or imprisonment. You're not looking your
best when you come out, but boy, you soon learn to cherish that
freedom. I swear that in a few weeks they actually looked happier,
you could just tell by the interest they showed in everything. They
were mindful chickens, and I've learned a lot from them. If you want
to be free, all you have to do is escape from your four-walled prisons
and possessions, and let go.

Lisa, forty-eight

There's a lot to be said for being free, although an illness can
place some limits on your freedom. The psychological tricks of the

advertising industry create a culture of chronic dissatisfaction and insecurity, to encourage us to strive for and buy stuff we don't need and then trap us into debt and the anxiety it brings. But what keeps us mentally and physically well has very little to do with ownership or material gain. You need some money to thrive and survive, and if you have the misfortune of serious illness, then the right piece of equipment can make all the difference. But whatever your state of health, it's often possible to live well if you're able to build good relationships, appreciate the present and get pleasure from small things. Money won't satisfy your mind, but CLANGERS can.

Getting a Grip on Your Habits

We all get stuck in our comfort zone, but bad habits can harm and kill us. Conversely, good habits don't always come easily. Sometimes, life can seem so meaningless and empty that we fill it with self-destructive behaviours. We all need passions to give us a purpose to live. But you can also be passionate about a fascinating job, and yet be so busy and engrossed by it, you have no time to look after yourself and eventually slip into bad habits. From September 2006 to April 2014, Sir David Nicholson was in charge of the English NHS, the most important and powerful person in a service employing 1.3 million people and focused on improving health. During that time he was knighted for services to the NHS, developed appalling health habits and didn't realize he was ill. He just fell into the trap of working ridiculous hours, getting the job done, overeating the wrong food, ignoring symptoms and staying in denial.

You might expect the most powerful man in the NHS to know the risks and recognize the symptoms of Type 2 diabetes in himself, particularly given that this often preventable disease accounts for a huge chunk of the NHS budget. But there's a big gap between knowing about something and acting on it. Many doctors don't practise what we preach. And you never know precisely what an illness will feel like until you've felt it. I sat at home with meningitis once, which luckily turned out to be viral rather than bacterial, or I might not be here now. A very experienced doctor I know sat on a burst appendix because, although he knew all the symptoms and signs of appendicitis, it just didn't feel like he was expecting it to feel. Other doctors I know have sat at home with 'heartburn' that turned out to be a heart attack. We can't always diagnose ourselves accurately, let alone you. Often it's a relative who forces us to face reality. If someone you love is worried about you, it's a big red flag to seek help. David Nicholson finally realized he had to get a grip on his health and lifestyle, and change for life. And he had a strong purpose in doing so – to be there for his family.

INSIDE THE HEAD OF THE NHS
'FOR YEARS MY LIFESTYLE WAS COMPLETELY AND UTTERLY UNHEALTHY'

Sir David Nicholson's Story

I just knew something was wrong with me. For several months I had been becoming increasingly, unusually tired and was needing to go to the toilet five or six times a night. I knew it wasn't overwork or stress but didn't know what it could be. My wife Sarah-Jane thought I was just a bit run down. This was towards the end of 2012. However, the travelling involved in being chief executive of the NHS, the birth of my daughter Rosa that November and the fact that I'd just moved house meant I didn't get round to seeing my GP until Christmas Eve, a while after the symptoms appeared. Pretty much right away my GP said, 'It sounds like diabetes to me.' He took some blood, put it into a machine and it showed that my blood glucose level was way beyond what it should be. That confirmed that I had Type 2 diabetes.

He said, 'You're going to the toilet a lot as your kidneys are responding to high levels of sugar in your blood and your body deals with that by urinating it out.' I said, 'Can I be cured? Can I get out of this?' But he said, 'No, you've got it for life.' He also explained that the main complications of diabetes are heart failure, stroke, kidney failure, blindness and amputation of a lower limb. I knew all that already; I'd given evidence to the public accounts committee about diabetes a few months earlier, ironically. But to hear a doctor saying this to me about me was sobering and very scary.

It was particularly sobering because my father, who'd been a plasterer, died when he was sixty-eight from emphysema and asthma. He spent his last years in a wheelchair. My grandfather, a labourer in a brass factory, also died in his sixties, of heart failure. So I'd always assumed I would die early too; that I wouldn't make seventy. My expectations were for no longer than that. It may sound weird but I was quite fatalistic about that. Unconsciously I wasn't looking after my health because I thought that's what would happen. My sons Liam and Paul from my first marriage are in their twenties. I'd always assumed I'd see them grow up. But this diagnosis of diabetes really made me realize that I might not be there for my little girl, Rosa.

The GP said to me, 'You have to think about the next twenty years and managing your condition.' I suddenly thought, Oh Lord. I always knew having a child when you're older – I was fifty-seven when she was born – meant there was the potential to not be around for much of their life. But suddenly the time I might have began to constrict in front of my eyes. I wasn't thinking, 'I might only be around until Rosa's twenty,' because, from what the GP said about my lifestyle and the blood sugar levels I had, the chances were that it would be much less than twenty years.

That's quite hard to hear: the diagnosis, then the complications, and then 'by the way it's your fault'. But in truth, it was absolutely, completely my fault. I had lost control of my health and my lifestyle. I had essentially abdicated responsibility for my own health and allowed it to get out of control, even though I was the chief executive of the NHS. The irony of that was huge, I know, not least because I used to stand on stage regularly and talk about health and healthcare. In all that time only one person pointed out to me the dissonance between what I was saying and what they saw on stage. The way I dealt with that dissonance was to say to myself, 'Yeah but I'm healthy, I'm fine, I'm not off sick, I'm robust.'

But I was deluding myself; completely deluding myself. That's why they call diabetes the silent killer. You can live with it for many years and not know you've got it; because you don't feel ill all the time, yet all these changes to your body are going on. It doesn't involve pain, or growths, or chemotherapy or anything like that, but it kills people, just like cancer. It's just not obvious to people that you've got it. In fact there are three times as many diabetics as people with cancer.

For years my lifestyle was completely and utterly unhealthy. My jobs in the NHS meant I was away from home a lot; three, four or even five nights a week. Every morning in the hotel I'd have bacon, egg, sausage, tomato and fries for breakfast, then there'd be a dinner most nights. I was at railway stations and motorway service stations a lot and would buy a triple-decker sandwich, muffin and bag of crisps – instant gratification, really. I'd always worked hard but after I separated from my first wife in 2001 I became obsessed with work, worked twenty-four/seven and was never off-duty.

I didn't think about the implications until I began growing out of all my clothes. Thank heaven for Marks and Spencer's elasticated-waist trousers. They allow massive self-deception and are a great boon to anyone who's putting on weight. I bought them with a thirty-eight or forty-inch waist, but they expanded, so I could kid myself that my weight wasn't as gross as it was, but actually it was. When I saw the GP that Christmas Eve I weighed 111 kilogrammes – seventeen stone and six pounds.

Looking back, I had been in denial. I couldn't quite see how that could have happened, because in my own mind I was significantly lighter than that. So that was quite a shock, how big I'd become. But it had happened over time. I'd not perceived any change. And I'd never, ever weighed myself. While I'm quite reflective about things I do, I was never really reflective about what I looked like. When the GP said, 'You've got diabetes,' I appreciated right away how serious and life-changing that was. I realized I had to get a grip on my lifestyle and resolved to take control of my health. I knew that if I really, really organized myself I could do it.

I completely overhauled my diet. I began to understand about and use low-GI foods, such as basmati rice and wholegrain bread, and also have brown bread, brown rice and brown pasta instead of their white equivalents. That made a massive difference to my glucose levels. Some diabetics get a little machine and a set of strips which you use when you do a little blood test on yourself four times a day, to check your glucose levels. You look at your score and you fill it in a book so you can see the trajectory of it. I used the targets for what my glucose levels should be as a motivational tool. When you do your blood test before a meal the number should be below seven, but if you do it two hours after you've eaten it needs to be below ten, because it goes up when you eat and then goes down again. So I saw the impact that eating certain things at certain times had on my numbers.

I've cut out almost all sauces. I've learned portion control is vital. For example, I now measure out the amount of pasta I should be eating, which turns out to be about a quarter of the amount I used to eat. Previously if Sarah-Jane hadn't finished her food I'd eat that too. I've stopped that. I'm more demanding in restaurants. I say, 'Don't put chips on the plate, as that's temptation,' or 'No butter, just plain as it is.'

I now eat grilled fish and don't eat too much bread. I don't have starters and eat nothing in between meals except maybe a little bag of tomatoes, chopped peppers or cucumbers. One of the reasons I decided to tell people I had diabetes was that if you're out eating with people and someone says, 'Have the chips,' if you say you're trying to lose weight they say, 'Oh go on, have them anyway,' whereas if I say I have diabetes they don't. In a strange way, people are much more supportive of you if they think you've got a disease you are tackling rather than dieting.

You see the same thing when people say, 'Have another pint.' I was brought up from the age of fourteen to think that on Friday night it's eight pints of bitter, and did that through my forties and into my fifties. Every Friday night I'd go out and have seven or eight pints. But I've now cut out beer altogether. Previously I would have an alcoholic drink of some sort three nights out of four. Now I have two small glasses of red wine twice a week. So I've undergone a dramatic revolution in my lifestyle. I've lost about three stone and am doing my best to keep my weight down.

Despite that I am now one of about 3.2 million people in the UK who have been diagnosed with diabetes. Some 225,000 more are diagnosed every year. Another 600,000 or so with Type 2 are still undiagnosed, so the real total is about 3.8 million. Ninety per cent of diabetics have Type 2, which is associated with lifestyle and obesity, whereas Type 1 is an autoimmune condition. It already costs the NHS about £10 billion, about 10 per cent of the budget. Diabetes UK says it will be 17 per cent of the budget within a generation. When I visited a hospital in Birmingham a few months ago I found 28 per cent of the inpatients had diabetes. Specialist diabetes doctors say that's pretty typical. It's clearly a huge and growing burden on the NHS.

So diabetes is a terrifying phenomenon as well as a horrible disease. It's incurable and life-limiting. It's also actually quite easy to get, as I discovered. As a country we need to have a wake-up call about diabetes. But it's also something we can and should do much more to prevent and help people manage it better when they get it. If we can tackle diabetes we will reduce the number of heart attacks and strokes related to diabetes, which is involved in about 24,000 early deaths a year in England and Wales, and also reduce the 6,000 lower limb amputations that happen every year, about 80 per cent of which are preventable. It's the complications of diabetes rather than the diabetes itself that kills people.

To prevent it and manage it, whole families need to change the way they eat and live. We need to promote healthy living and make that easier. We need easier access to primary care to help ensure earlier diagnosis. Much more money should go into the Expert Patient Programme, which helps people manage their condition. I found that very useful. Greater use of education, technology and social psychology would help, too.

But people also need to take control of their own health, as I've now done, irrespective of whether they're diabetic or not. It is possible to change, though that's rarely easy. Partners are vital, too. If the spouse of someone with diabetes says, 'I'm going to keep on eating chips and cake and pie and you can sit opposite me with a lettuce leaf,' that's not going to work. It's good for partners too when these sorts of changes happen. I'm now our family shopper. We all only eat what I buy. My wife's discovered brown bread and has lost weight too and is happy about that. I am now much more confident

about seeing my daughter Rosa grow up. I think I have done
everything I can to make sure that our relationship goes on as long
as possible. I hope that by managing my diabetes as best I can I am
extending my life. I really want to be around for as long as I can.

(Full article appeared in *The Guardian*, 16 May 2014
Reproduced with DN's permission)

We like to think of themselves as indestructible, but we all get ill.
Sometimes the symptoms of illness come on suddenly and severely,
sometimes they creep up gradually. Often they've been brewing and
rusting away for many years without us noticing or trying to stop them
in their tracks. Kidney disease, lung disease, liver disease, heart disease, vascular disease and diabetes can all be silent killers. One way to
slow them down is to avoid the addiction of workaholism, if you're
lucky enough to have a job, and to live a more balanced life full of
CLANGERS. It's not easy in the NHS, because the demand seems
limitless and time is always limited. Sadly, the mental and physical
health of people working in the NHS is very poor, and 700,000 are
overweight or obese (i.e. ordinary humans struggling to stay afloat in
modern Britain).

David Nicholson's story shows how it is possible to replace bad habits with good ones, but it took the shock of a serious diagnosis to
change his mind-set and get him to focus on what really mattered to
him (being there for his family). His achievement in getting fit, eating
well, losing weight and controlling his diabetes without the need for
drugs matches anything he achieved while running the NHS. But he
found it very hard to do both at the same time. The roots of many
physical illnesses lie in mental health. The brain can only deal with so
much stress before it spreads out into the body. Bad habits are often an
emotional response to an unhappy, pressurized, chaotic life. But
humans are also extraordinarily resilient. They bounce back. The one
thing you can say about your darkest days is that you survived them.
And if you learn to harness the power of your mind to improve your
mood, it can make a huge difference to your health, and your ability to
get the right healthcare for you.

A lot of it comes down to replacing bad habits with good ones. A recovering alcoholic turns the habit of never refusing a drink into never accepting one. A family may get into the habit of never buying sweetened drinks, or never having them at mealtimes. If you eat out a lot, you can get into the habit of never having bread or only ever eating half a pudding. In time, these small changes make a big difference.

So it is with seeing a doctor. You can replace the bad habit of never asking any questions to the good (and realistic) habit of always asking three, i.e. 'What is the most likely diagnosis? What else could it be? How would I know?' The more you get into the habit of asking questions, the easier it gets. And research in the field of positive psychology has shown you can even learn daily habits to improve your happiness.

Happiness Habits – Using Your Mind to Improve Your Mood

Anxiety and low mood are very common among patients with chronic diseases and their carers, and mental illness also puts you at higher risk of physical illness. Confidence, courage and optimism are crucial to mental health, and although very severe mental illness needs prompt drug treatment and specialist care, other illnesses can be helped by psychotherapy, cognitive therapy, mindfulness, acceptance and commitment therapy and positive psychology. These approaches can be very helpful in understanding your past, coping with illness in the present and with the complex choices that need to be made in negotiating the NHS. Your mood is like a horse, with your mind as the rider. You'll never completely learn to control it but you can learn to accept it, live well with it and jump over the bars you set for yourself. Crucial to this is learning that the brain is quite plastic (so called 'neuroplasticity'), so what you focus on is what grows. Happiness has less to do with our circumstances, and more to do with our interpretation of those circumstances, which we at least have some control over. Miriam Akhtar is a positive psychologist who herself suffers from depression and has learned how to use her mind to improve her mood.

'WHAT YOU FOCUS ON IS WHAT GROWS'

Miriam Akhtar's Story

Of all the relationships I've been in, one of the longest lasting was with the 'black dog' of depression. Mild, moderate or major – I've experienced them all. Now it's rare for me to feel low and when I do dip down I bounce back fast. I have learnt how to keep the blues at bay – naturally – and developed my capacity for happiness.

Mine is not an unusual story. Every life has its ups and downs. Depression has a variety of causes; in my case what happened is that a pretty average childhood came to a sudden and brutal conclusion when my father collapsed and died. I was ten years old. Not long afterwards I went through the transition from junior to senior school. Life had changed radically in a short space of time and I felt the clouds gathering to block out the innocent sunshine of youth. I coped by becoming a teen workaholic. This was a successful strategy for many years and I did well in education and in my career. I had, though, a curious habit of interrupting positive experiences by asking, 'But am I happy?' And in an instant the happiness would evaporate.

I had always imagined that by the millennium I would be in a loving partnership with two children. But even though I went into my thirties in a relationship, a break-up led to me morphing into a singleton. Every birthday I wondered if this was the year that things would change but there were already clues that family life might not be my fate. Just like Bridget Jones, the eponymous single girl, I had a creative job in an industry where over 50 per cent of women aged thirty-plus do not have children. When you're married to the job it's very easy to miss out on the landmarks in life that we all take for granted, like children. I took a sabbatical to deal with the Big Question that all singletons face. If I don't have children, then what am I going to do with my life?

Taking time out turned out to be a bad idea because it gave me too much space to dwell on what was wrong. Those grey clouds that had dogged me throughout life were gathering again. I usually suppressed them by throwing myself into yet another new project but this time I spiralled downwards. The doctor diagnosed depression and wrote a prescription for anti-depressants.

I ended up trying three types of anti-depressants but none of them worked for me and their side effects left me feeling worse. I went into therapy but all that did was to put me in touch with my deepest pain. It didn't make me any happier. Talking about my long, dark night of the soul only served to keep me in that long, dark night. Like Bridget Jones I reached for the self-help books but it felt like I was faking a happy smile to mask the undercurrent of despair.

The turning point came one morning when I noticed a funny smell coming from the dishwasher. Rank water was building up inside. Feeling bluer than blue, I thrashed around with some tools until a pipe burst and disaster – the kitchen flooded. Defeated I sat there on the damp floor and wailed. I'd spent months focusing on how bad I was feeling and where had it got me – to a sky-high bill for calling out the emergency plumber. I'd exhausted all the usual ways of dealing with depression, none of which were working for me. I was going to have to find my own road to recovery.

I'd first come across positive psychology in the mid-nineties before its official birth as a new branch of psychology. I was intrigued to discover that there was a 'science' of happiness, that psychologists were applying the scientific method to investigate the characteristics of wellbeing as it had been applied previously to study mental disorders and illness. It made a lot of sense to me. Here at last was evidence-based knowledge on how to develop our capacity for happiness. My interest was sparked initially by a radio programme I was producing on the subject but over the next decade I applied my journalistic skills to investigate everything that was emerging from the new science of wellbeing. I devoured every book and research paper that I could get my hands on. Here was a goldmine of scientific knowledge that could make a substantial difference to human happiness.

Sitting there that day on the damp floor, I resolved to see how positive psychology might work for depression. So out went the therapy and the pills and instead of focusing on how low I was feeling I tried some of the techniques you'll find in my book. What happened was that slowly but surely I noticed that the darkness began to recede and there were more and more days on which the sun came out from behind the clouds. I found a way out of depression and as a bonus discovered my purpose in life – to help others onto that path to happiness. I found what gives me meaning in life and the breakthrough had come courtesy of a broken dishwasher!

I wanted to share the knowledge so I trained as a coach to put positive psychology into practice. Nothing gives me greater satisfaction than witnessing the change in clients as their capacity for happiness grows and their lives begin to flourish. The positive changes on the inside are often matched by positive changes on the outside. Many of my clients fear, like I once did, that they might be incapable of happiness, so it is wonderful to see their pleasure and surprise when they discover that positive psychology really does work – they feel better and life takes a turn for the better.

I wish positive psychology had been around when I was that small girl who suffered a trauma. The wellbeing of young people is something that remains close to my heart. I work with organizations that help vulnerable youngsters and am one of the trainers of the Penn Resilience Programme, which builds resilience in teenagers. Incidentally, it's never too late to master the techniques of positive psychology, even if you have spent a lifetime in a relationship with depression. It just takes practice. It worked for me – I now enjoy a much more sustainable happiness and wellbeing – and it can work for you too.

Learning From Miriam

Miriam's excellent book is called *Positive Psychology for Overcoming Depression*. I know her, admire her and wrote the Foreword. I feel like we're kindred spirits as she too lost her dad when she was young. Many people can learn to be happier by practising the habits of happiness, just as you can be healthier by developing healthy habits. Remember, our minds are remarkably plastic and continually developing. What you focus on is what grows. If you do what you're good at and what makes you happy, you're thankful for what you have and you thank those who help and support you, you're far more likely to be successful, content and happy. It's also worth doing CLANGERS on your own. If you can enjoy your own company, you can recover from most of what life throws at you.

The human brain evolved to accentuate the negative to avoid harm, and this negative thinking can be extremely helpful when you're under threat. When you're using the NHS, you have to use both positive and negative thinking to get the best care possible in the circumstances, to hope for the best but have a plan for the worst, and to temper your positivity with some safety-conscious observations and healthy scepticism.

Life can change very suddenly, and you have no idea how you will react when shit happens. But humans have evolved a remarkable ability to cope. Illness and death are part of life, and they happen to us all. The more we talk about them and share our experiences, the less frightening they become. Fear and frustration never vanish but we move on by accepting what we can't change and committing to changing things we still can, and that matter to most of us.

LIVING WITH RESTRICTION

All illnesses place restrictions on your life and, as people live longer, many are living for fifty years or more with incurable illnesses. The sense of grief and loss for any life-changing diagnosis should not be underestimated, but neither should the resilience and ingenuity of those who learn not just to come to terms with their illness – and the restrictions it imposes – but to live well with purpose and meaning, and to help others facing similar challenges. With a chronic disease you have to interact more with the NHS not just to get the right care, but to personalize the care around what matters to you.

To do this, you have to decide how much you want to reveal of yourself as a person, and to think about and say what it is you need help with.

It's particularly hard for rare diseases, which many doctors and nurses will only see once in a lifetime so you may be far more expert in all aspects of your illness than we are. But first you have to get the right diagnosis. Cancer is common – one in two of us will get it, one in three of us will die with it – and when it is suspected you are supposed to be seen by a specialist within two weeks. This system can work very well for common cancers, but rarer cancers can go for months without being diagnosed. When they are, it's essential that treatment occurs at a specialist centre that has the expertise, research and resources to give the best care. Even then, it's far from simple.

Rarer cancers such as neuro-endocrine tumours (NETs) can start with non-specific symptoms, and when they are diagnosed they can vary hugely in their grade and body site, so simple pathways of care rarely fit the bill and you need to get to a specialist centre with a comprehensive multidisciplinary team that has the experience of treating patients like you.

Due to late diagnosis, 90 per cent of patients with metastatic NETs cannot be cured. Data from the NET Patient Foundation (I'm a patron) suggests that 61 per cent of patients are diagnosed with the wrong disease prior to diagnosis. The most common wrong diagnosis is irritable bowel syndrome.

Like many great charities, the NET Patient Foundation sends patients a very informative video, patient literature and information on ways in which they can get referred to a specialist centre. They help with that process if needed. They have a wonderful online Q&A forum which allows your questions to be answered by specialists who know what they're talking about, getting you the right information and advice quickly. They have a NET Natter initiative which combines support groups all over the UK. Patients support each other and become in some cases quite powerful within the political arena. But even with charity support and specialist care, treatment is far from straightforward.

'I FEEL THE NEED TO TELL OTHER PATIENTS ABOUT MY EXPERIENCE'

Patrick's Story (aged forty-two)

After months of abdominal pains, incessant itching and erratic bowel movements, an ultrasound on my thirty-first birthday finally revealed the cause: a tumour at the head of my pancreas that was blocking my bile duct.

The immediate diagnosis of pancreatic cancer seemed too incredible to contemplate and even harder to explain to my parents, friends and in particular to my future wife, Helen, whose father was struggling with his lung cancer treatment at the time. Confined to my hospital bed, I saw brave faces but little of the worries that were definitely shared beyond the ward.

Instead, I discovered the treatment regimen that patients with pancreatic tumours have to follow. Nil by mouth (in my case this lasted some six weeks), a feeding tube up a vein from my elbow to my shoulder, two lots of ERCP (a procedure where a stand is inserted down your throat to release the flow of bile), followed by a biopsy with the world's biggest needle which would confirm my tumour was neuroendocrine cancer.

While the procedures relieved some of the symptoms, I soon realized that they were only making me better so that they could do something more drastic: remove most of my pancreas, some of my stomach and intestines and stick it all back together again in an operation called a Whipple. I was told that 4 per cent of patients who undergo the procedure die as a result, but that compared favourably, so the surgeon said, with my 100 per cent chance of death from the tumour if they didn't operate. The procedure would take at least seven hours if successful, so I was desperate to know the time when I woke. It'd been seven and a half hours; a significant success with the bulk of the cancer removed.

However, metastatic disease is a reality of neuroendocrine tumours. There is no concept of remission, no prospect of being disease-free (only free from the visible disease) and I had to clear lesions in the liver as well as some tumour at the edge of the surgical site that it hadn't been possible to cut out. So began a cycle of scans, follow-up appointments and treatment.

Firstly I injected myself with interferon three times a week. After eighteen months or so of flu-like symptoms I began to tolerate the side effects much better; the therapy was effective for almost three more years before my tumour started to grow again.

The next treatment was due to be Sunitinib, which a new research study had demonstrated to be very effective in a small cohort of patients. After several months of the Royal Free trying to obtain funding, I began to take the pills. I remember reading the sheet that explained the dosage, which unfurled to reveal several pages of side effects; my favourite being that it might cause extra tubes to grow in the gastrointestinal tract.

Sure enough, after just three doses my digestive system broke down and I ended up in hospital for a week, ironically not with any documented side effect, but with an ileus, a condition that it later transpired only one other patient who had taken Sunitinib had experienced. This is a particular issue with NETs: there are so few patients that it is difficult to predict either beneficial or detrimental effects with any certainty.

Next up: chemotherapy. The combination of three drugs shouldn't just have shrunk my tumour, it should also have relieved some of my symptoms. In the end it did neither. Eighty per cent of patients on this regime get some kind of benefit. I just happened to be one of the remaining 20 per cent. I was weak, nauseous and feverish and ended up in hospital again. After ten weeks of treatment, learning that the chemotherapy hadn't worked actually came as a relief: I really didn't want to continue. I was seriously underweight and unable to socialize or participate in any activities with my children.

I started physiotherapy and acupuncture, and made a concerted attempt to put on weight, which is no easy task when you've got very little pancreas. I then started to take Everolimus, albeit with some trepidation. It's a similar drug in many ways to the Sunitinib that I had taken and had landed me in hospital, and I was by no means fully recovered from the after-effects of the chemotherapy. I also started to inject myself with octreotide, a synthetic growth-inhibiting hormone. I was confident that I could follow the twice-daily injection routine, having previously injected myself with interferon for so long. But that wasn't the case. I found the injections painful and the consequent diarrhoea difficult to tolerate, so I quickly abandoned them. I persisted with the Everolimus, however, which to my surprise gave me relatively few problems and I recently discovered had a positive effect in beginning to control my cancer.

The litanies of treatments described above are by no means the full extent of the care I've received. I've had many forms of investigative procedures – some more invasive than others – and lots of other medication to help me tolerate the medicine that was supposed to treat cancer. At one point I was taking close to thirty doses of medication a day. I'll always need medication simply to eat, and have taken pancreatic enzymes with every meal for the last eleven years. But it's essential to point out that without the specialist care at the Royal Free most of this treatment simply wouldn't have been available. The undue focus on a cancer's primary location would mean my case would be completely misunderstood and as a consequence mistreated.

The work done by the NET Patient Foundation in educating clinicians about neuroendocrine tumours is crucial to ensuring that people like me have their cancer properly recognized and treated by people who understand and participate in the latest NET research.

Where does that leave me as a patient of some eleven years? Normal is very different, both for me and in particular for my wife. It's made up of hospital visits at least once a month and scans every three months, always uncertain of what the results will show. It's a life where tumour and treatments have combined to beat up my body in unexpected ways: whether weakening the muscles around my spine, or causing tooth decay, or huge variations in bowel movements, or simply making me too tired to spend time with the family, to work or to socialize.

Beyond the physical, you need to be highly pragmatic about your life, particularly financially. Planning for when there is no income, whether temporarily or permanently, is a major concern. Being self-employed may seem like an unnecessary burden, but I've first-hand experience of how difficult employers make life for staff who have long-term illnesses. Running my own company gives me a sense of control that I have very little of in the rest of my life.

There's also the matter of privacy. I did an interview about NETs to the BBC a few years ago. What do you tell clients about that? Or business partners? Or parents at school? And what do you tell your children? What do you tell a seven-year-old about why you can't get out of bed or why you need to stay in hospital? What do you tell a three-year-old?

I feel the need to tell other patients about my experience in the hope they'll benefit, ready to ask more questions and approach what will be unpleasant experiences with a little more knowledge and a little less fear. And I want to tell people who can influence how our treatment is delivered so that they can help all patients to access the best services.

Beyond that, I'll keep my cancer to myself and the people who help me to deal with it.

Learning From Patrick

Patrick's story is another of huge courage in the face of a deeply unpleasant and disruptive disease, a desire to share his story to help others and a demonstration of how much patients can learn to participate in complex decisions about their care and administer powerful drugs and treatments to themselves with the right training. Asking the right questions is key to living with fear, access to specialist care is essential for the right treatment and you need to feel part of a team and always kept in the loop. But even at the best units, treatment is not guaranteed to succeed.

With knowledge, skills and courage, it is possible for seriously ill patients to transform their lives by treating themselves at home. It takes time, training and teamwork, but why accept a limited life when a much freer one could be yours? People can be trained and trusted to do their own kidney dialysis at home.

'IF YOU CAN DO YOUR OWN DIALYSIS, YOU CAN DO ANYTHING.'

Stuart's Story
I've met patients with kidney failure who were previously having to travel to hospital three times a week for dialysis, which is very

disruptive to family and work life, but then they were trained to do it at home. For Stuart, and his wife Lynn, it wasn't easy. Stuart had to learn to stick needles into a special 'shunt' in his arm, and they had to be well organized and safety conscious to take control and responsibility for a complicated machine that is keeping Stuart alive. But they got lots of training and support from their specialist nurse, and it transformed their lives. As Stuart put it:

'It's not just the time saved going to and from hospital, it's that you can vary the time you do your dialysis to fit in with family outings and special times. It's also meant that I've been able to take on more work, and provide for my family and pay a bit more into a pension which is very important to me. I actually feel better, and my blood readings are better than they were in hospital. But I think the biggest bonus has been improving my self-confidence. I never thought I'd be able to do this, but we have. We've learned a lot more about my disease. And it's also made me realize if I can take control over my dialysis, I can take more control over anything. I've become better with my fluid intake and diet and other health issues, and I can get access to all my blood results from my computer as soon as they are ready. As well as confidence, it's given me power and control and independence, which are three things that kidney failure had taken away from me. I've even taught myself to play the guitar while I'm dialysing at home, something I wouldn't dare to have done at hospital. If you can do your own dialysis, you can do anything.'

Not every patient or carer is willing or able to take on more responsibility for self-care and treatment, but if you are – and you get the right support and training – even life-threatening illnesses can be a little less restricting. And the effect on your confidence and self-esteem can be huge.

We can all learn new knowledge, skills and courage and we can all share it and pass it on. We can all surprise ourselves with what we can do. I've chaired hundreds of conferences in the last twenty-five years and heard hundreds of speakers. There are some that have changed the way I look at the world and how I practise medicine. One is Clare Bowen, an ordinary working mum who lost her daughter and husband in the most tragic circumstances and has risen to become an inspirational patient safety leader. We'll come to her story later (page 226). Another is Miles Hilton-Barber, 'a very ordinary man who happens to be blind'. He is also a pilot, polar explorer, desert explorer, scuba diver, extreme marathon runner, grand prix driver, sky diver, white-water rafter, bob-sleigher, shark cager, etc.

'IF A BLIND BLOKE CAN DO ALL THIS, WHAT ARE YOU WAITING FOR?'

Miles Hilton-Barber's Story

'Who would have thought a hundred years ago that anyone could fly? And who would have thought a hundred years on that a blind man would fly as well? Technology is amazing, isn't it?'

I don't quite buy the 'ordinary bloke' tag but Miles is an extremely funny, modest, down-to-earth, inspirational and slightly dangerous speaker. Not all of his wild exploring goes to plan, but he gets it back on track with great tenacity and spirit. His achievements could teach the NHS a huge amount about the importance of resilience, good humour, teamwork, safety and technology. But his message for individuals is even stronger. If a blind bloke can do all this, what are you waiting for? As he told a convention of other blind people:

'I'm just like one beggar telling another beggar where to find a square meal. Do you understand what I am saying? I am just telling you guys where it's at. It's for you to go and grab it.'

Miles speaks with such authenticity and warmth, you can't fail to be moved. And his metaphors for surviving and thriving are very strong.

'There are two quotes that have meant a lot in my life. One is a Danish proverb that says that "Life does not consist in holding a good hand of cards, but in playing a poor hand well." I wasted years of my life when I heard that I was going to become blind; I thought I couldn't live my dreams, I couldn't have any big goals in life. Now I realize that, if we just play the hand of cards we have been given, it is enough for us to do anything we want with our lives. Play your hand of cards as well as you can!

'The other is a quote from Lawrence of Arabia, one of my great heroes. In his book *The Seven Pillars of Wisdom* he says this: "All men dream dreams, but not all men dream equally, for there are those who dream at night in the empty recesses of their minds, and they awake in the morning to find that, behold, it was just a dream. But there are other men and women who are dangerous dreamers. [I love that – dangerous dreamers] For these are men and women who dream in the daytime with their eyes open, that they might fulfil their dreams." So don't be a daydreamer, be a dangerous dreamer. The only limits in our lives are those we accept ourselves.'

I've heard Miles speak several times, and get a standing ovation on each occasion, and he inspires me because he simply refuses to be labelled or limited by his blindness. His card, which I keep stuck up in my office, is a photo of him in scuba gear with a white stick, proudly pushing his friend Mike, a double leg amputee paralysed from the chest down, in a wheelchair across the floor of the Red Sea. It makes me smile and lifts my spirits whenever I leave the house. As Miles puts it:

'Attitude is critical for success. As long as you are pointing in the right direction, every step counts.'

3

Getting the Right Care for You

THE RIGHT MIND-SET FOR THE NHS

*It's as important to know what sort of person has the disease
as to know what sort of disease the person has.*
Caleb Parry, doctor, 1755–1822

There are two reasons for using the NHS. The first is because you've been invited and the second is because you, or someone near you, thinks you need to. If you feel well but you've been invited for a health check or screening, it's entirely up to you whether you go. You shouldn't be pressured or coerced into attending. There is no right or wrong answer – it simply depends on how medicalized you want your life to be and whether you want to be at slightly lower risk of a disease you may already be at low risk of.

Medicine works by making a diagnosis or risk assessment and offering a choice of treatments that should help you improve, prolong or restore your quality of life. Never lose sight of that goal. There is also a downside to diagnosis – you pick up a disease label and may have to fight not to be defined by it – so make sure there's a good chance that you will benefit before you subject yourself to screening, health checks, tests and treatments. 'How likely am I to benefit from this?' should always follow 'what is most likely to happen if we did nothing?'

A surprising number of symptoms – perhaps 50 per cent – are 'medically unexplained' and don't lead to a diagnosis or treatment. How we live our lives often defeats medical science, and although many symptoms do get better in time, they're more likely to get better by living gentler lives and getting a good balance of thinking, being and doing, rather than being slaves to a job or lifestyle. Doing CLANGERS every day may work better for you than any drug.

Treatments can be life-saving and life-enhancing, but a surprising number operate at the fringes, offering marginal benefit at best and merely serving to make well people anxious about their new disease or risk label (pre-diabetes, pre-hypertension, pre-death). You should never be defined or diminished by a diagnostic label. You are never epileptic, but you may be an artist, mother, sister, daughter, runner, dog-lover, gardener and cake-baker who just happens to have epilepsy. The NHS is trying to move to personalized care where people are no longer referred to as 'the diabetic in bed seven', but in order to personalize your care, you have to share part of your life and what matters to you with the people caring for you.

Mental illness can be very stigmatizing, and the emotional pain it causes can be just as severe, if not more so, than physical pain. However, at present nearly two in three people who have mental illnesses do not get any treatment, and some of the treatment that is available is based on poor evidence. For example, drug companies have got very rich on spreading the myth that depression is caused by low levels of serotonin but the evidence to support this is poor. Psychological therapies such as CBT do work, as do drugs for severe illness, but given that nearly 40 per cent of all illness in the UK is mental illness, it gets far too little recognition and funding. And it's hard to be assertive and seek out the care you need when you're anxious or depressed (and often both). The NHS has a programme called IAPT (Improving Access to Psychological Therapies), which has made good progress, and websites have been developed to provide online support and learning on how to keep your mind healthy (e.g. www.minded.org.uk/) The 'U Can Cope' campaign also offers excellent advice and support. And the Samaritans are always there (08457 90 90 90).

Sexually transmitted diseases sound horrible, sexually transmitted infections a little less so. Sexually shared infections are a more accurate description that has yet to catch on. 'Herpes' retains a ridiculous power to shock and frighten for something that's usually just a cold sore gone south or chicken pox on your privates. Words are how we change the world and medical language needs to be efficient and accurate under pressure, but words can also cause enormous harm. When you use the NHS, brace yourself that not only may some of your tests be 'abnormal' but you may even be described as abnormal or an extension of your illness. Don't allow it. Always remember you are normal for you, and don't let anyone else tell you otherwise. If you need comedic inspiration read *What the **** Is Normal?!* by the wonderfully normal Francesca Martinez.

Learning to Swim

Falling ill is a bit like falling in a river. You might wander too close to the edge and slip in, you might dive in and be damned, or you might even be pushed in. Or you might just find yourself in the water with no warning and not sure how you got there. It can be sudden or gradual, very unlucky and very unfair. Illness and injury can happen to any of us at any time. The shock of falling in can lead to numbness, anger, denial and confusion. But when you're ready, you need to stop treading water and learn how to swim.

Learning to be a more active patient, like learning to swim, needs knowledge, skills and courage. But once you've cracked it, it stays with you for life. You may in time become a confident swimmer, but it's hard to be confident when you're frightened and out of control. I've seen many supremely confident people – business men and women, lawyers, politicians, journalists, even other doctors – lose it all when they get seriously ill. It takes real courage to find your voice and speak up for yourself as a patient or carer. You may have to overcome fatigue, brain fog, fears about your illness and any anxieties you might have about the quality of your care. It's like being thrown in the deep end without ever having had a swimming lesson.

When I first walked onto an NHS ward in 1984, many patients were discouraged from being active partners in their care. Some were not even told if they had a serious diagnosis such as cancer, multiple sclerosis or dementia. We assumed you weren't able to contribute, didn't want to know or that telling you might just make you more anxious and unable to cope. And doctors didn't have to waste emotion and energy on those difficult conversations about death and disability. But not knowing your diagnosis meant that you couldn't possibly participate in important decisions about your care, involve your loved ones or plan properly for the future. Too often we just left you silently adrift in the water, while we tried to figure out a way of getting you back to the river bank or gently out to sea. We might not even tell you which direction you were heading. We pretended to do the worrying for you, and left you to figure it out for yourself.

So patients taught themselves to swim. I remember dressing up in an infection control 'space suit' to 'greet' the first patients I had met with HIV. Ignorance, prejudice, stigma and blame abounded, nobody wanted to get in the water alongside them, and many extraordinarily brave people died before their time. Other brave patients pretty soon learned how to swim. They learned everything they could possibly learn about HIV, they shared knowledge, skills and courage, they knew where all the trials for new drugs were taking place, they read the latest research the minute it was published and they demanded the best care. They knew it was a race against the clock.

Today, if you're lucky enough to live in a country that can afford the drugs, HIV is a chronic disease rather than an early death sentence. It's no picnic, it can't currently be cured but you can live long and well with it (and you can often avoid it with condoms or clean needles). Drug companies, NHS staff and amazingly dedicated research scientists deserve huge credit, but it would not have happened nearly so quickly if these brave patients and their carers hadn't become such powerful swimmers. Respectful collaboration in a team where people on both sides share knowledge, skills and courage, and are unafraid to challenge, to raise concerns, to disagree, and to love and laugh together is where the greatest NHS care and strongest swimmers are born.

Humans often take the path of least resistance, and when you're ill, it's usually easiest to lie back and let the professionals get on with it. But if you have an illness for life, there comes a time when you need to get more involved and to share what matters most to you so your care can be built around that. Remember though that there is no right way to be a patient. Different approaches work for different people.

'LISTEN TO ME, LEARN FROM ME AND EARN MY TRUST'

First, it's my body, my mind and my data. I may not know all the fancy anatomical terms, nor fully how things work, but I can often tell you when they're not working, so please treat me as a person not a body part. And let me have control of my medical records. Medicine divides me into systems – heart, brain, eyes, kidneys, etc – none of them work in isolation. You need my help to join up my care. I have diabetes, and I don't care where my flu vaccine, medicines or blood meter come from, I just want the right care for me, delivered safely, kindly and quickly, and the people supporting me to work in a seamless way. Second, I'm paying for the NHS, and I'm going to get more and more demanding as I begin to understand the system better. I'll soon be given my own budget to spend on my healthcare, so work with me in partnership. Third, I'm the one who has to live with the condition twenty-four/seven: to monitor my blood sugar, to make the changes to my doses, to try to remember to take the medicine, to eat better, to constantly be aware of this blot on my copybook. To help me, I want the NHS to truly engage with me as a customer. Give me information, give me time, help set and manage my expectations, train me to better help myself and therefore the whole NHS. Listen to me, learn from me and earn my trust. You are, or all too soon will be, one of us one day.

Mark Duman, passionate about patient empowerment

We all raise the bar on our NHS care in different ways. Demanding better information, support and training about diabetes is one way, taking time to get to know the staff treating you and building good relationships is another. One of the biggest frustrations for people using the NHS is the lack of continuity. It's very hard to build relationships with the staff when you rarely see the same person twice, and – exasperating though it is – you often need to repeat your story. The NHS and social care computer systems should link up but they don't, and the staff treating you may have vital gaps in their knowledge about you. Carrying a printed copy of your medical records with you containing all the key information (your current problems, past medical history, investigations, drugs, allergies and copies of key letters) can make a huge difference.

The internet is revolutionizing healthcare because it gives you instant access to information, support, tips and tactics that previous patients simply didn't have. Information is like a drug – it can be very beneficial but also harmful, especially if it is wrong or the dose is too high. The safest option is to stick to accredited, official health sites but if you wander a little off piste you can find inspiration and ideas from patients all over the world who've set up their own websites and blogs to share their experiences. The experience of one patient may not apply to you, or it may ring bells with you and give you confidence and courage. Here are some of my favourite examples of motivational advice from people who know what it is to live, thrive and survive with serious illness.

LEARNING FROM PATIENT LEADERS

There is no such thing as a stupid question. Often when we're first diagnosed with a serious or chronic illness, we don't even know what questions to ask. Learn what you can from trusted sources; talking to other patients can also be extremely beneficial. To be empowered, we must be educated, and to be educated we must understand all our options. Your doctor is the medical expert, but you are the expert when it comes to your body. I heed the words of a prominent oncologist who once said, 'When you gather all of the information, questions tend to answer themselves.'

AnneMarie Ciccarella, fifty-seven, diagnosed with invasive lobular breast cancer in July 2006; blogs at chemobrainfog.com

My doctor is a diabetes expert, but I am the leading expert in my diabetes. My opinion and preferences are just as important as those of my healthcare team, and working together with my doctor to create a personalized approach in managing my Type 1 diabetes has earned me the best health outcomes.

Kerry Sparling, thirty-five, diagnosed with Type 1 diabetes in 1986; blogs about it at sixuntilme.com

Speak up! The most important lesson I've learned about being an empowered patient is to share my story with others. By raising my voice and sharing my health experiences, others are enlightened about how they too can take charge of their own healthcare and improve their own quality of life. By not being silent, I've forged better relationships with my doctors, who are now able to better meet my healthcare needs.

Tiffany Peterson, twenty-eight, a lupus e-Patient
advocate who hosts frequent #LupusChat events on Twitter

Patients and their loved ones must make the commitment to invest a small amount of time and energy in educating themselves about their condition and about patient safety issues and strategies. There are many simple actions that patients can take to ensure they receive safe medical care and to function as true members of their healthcare teams . . . Patients who have the ability to work in partnership with their providers as full team members will experience safer and more satisfying outcomes. Once they possess the right information and skillset, empowered patients will be the largest, most cost-effective grass-roots healthcare lobbying group in history.

Julia Hallisy, fifty-one, spent years advocating
for her daughter Kate, who was diagnosed with
bilateral retinoblastoma at five months old; Kate fought
the cancer, which starts in the retina, five times by age
ten, and ultimately lost her battle with the disease in 2000

I've created the acronym HEALING as a reminder of my favourite tips. It has helped me receive excellent care and improved health outcomes:

H A Health summary is vital. List conditions, medicines, doctors, interventions, etc.

E Become the 'Expert' in you! Research your disease, medications and alternative therapies.

A Accept support; having a health advocate is crucial during emergencies.

L Look for a second opinion if necessary.

I Involve yourself. Most doctors appreciate patients who collaborate and take an active role in their care.

N Say 'No!' when something doesn't feel right.

G Give thanks to good medical providers. 'Thank you' can make all the difference.

Marisa Zeppieri-Caruana, thirty-six, of LupusChick.com

I was diagnosed with multiple sclerosis in the spring of 2005 and have since learned many lessons about living well with a chronic illness. The most important lesson I have learned, however, is to be your own advocate. No one knows you better than you. In order to be the best possible advocate for yourself, you need to educate yourself on your disease, as well as the ins and outs of the healthcare system. Research doctors and therapists who can help you, communicate openly and effectively with your healthcare providers, and most importantly – never give up hope. You are worth fighting for!

Matt Cavallo, thirty-eight, was fully functioning and healthy when he went numb from the waist down and lost the ability to walk, leading to a multiple sclerosis diagnosis at age twenty-eight

Sometimes it feels like the healthcare system is designed to disempower you. When you're sitting in a hospital room in a thin gown that barely covers you, discussing your health – a most precious thing – you're at your most vulnerable. PatientsLikeMe members know that by connecting with other patients who have travelled the road ahead, they can learn about the choices, what to expect and how to meet doctors as equals. They know their voice is the most important thing in reaching the right decisions. The best care happens when patients use the collective expertise of other patients' experiences. So connect with others like you to become an expert on your own health and find your voice. The next time you have to wear that gown, you'll feel a little less naked.

Ben Heywood, forty-two, president and director of PatientsLikeMe, an online network for people with chronic conditions; he and his brother Jamie were inspired to found the company in 2004 by their brother Stephen's battle with amyotrophic lateral sclerosis, or ALS

In 2004, I was diagnosed with a rare form of lymphoma with a prognosis of only a few months. I had never dealt with anything so difficult and just went along with everything I was told by the oncologist, just short of starting chemo. To this day I don't know why, but I decided to get a second opinion before consenting to treatment. Turned out I didn't have cancer after all. So the most important lesson I can share is to be fully engaged in every medical decision you must make, create decision-points yourself and always get a second opinion if your recommended treatment is invasive, toxic or long term.

Tricia Torrey, a sixty-something patient advocate and author of *Every Patient's Advocate*

I'm sixty-four. In the sixties I learned that step one of empowerment is to know what you want. Step two is consciousness raising: realize who's saying what to whom, and what assumptions that might imply. Perhaps it's what you'd like; if not, step three is to ask for it. Enlightened patients (and clinicians) know that nobody knows everything – neither patient nor clinician – and approach it as a partnership, in what we call 'participatory medicine.'

Dave deBronkart, cancer survivor, e-Patient Dave, blogger and activist

Some British patients feel guilty about seeking out and asking for the right care, because they worry it might deprive others of the care they need. In fact, if you can improve your chances of getting the right care for you, it is far more likely to be successful and to save the NHS money for others. The right care is usually a lot cheaper than the wrong care.

How you seek the right care for you is also critical. Aggression never works and assertiveness is often more effective with a bit of humour. The

NHS is not coping easily with the demands placed on it, so delays are inevitable and you need to take as much responsibility as you can for sorting yourself out. There are some excellent apps and text systems such as Buddy and Flo to help you. They use text message prompts, support and diaries to give you more control, keep your care on track and remind you of the changes you need to make in your life. And when you do get the right care and get better, you can share your experiences and tips so others can learn how you did it, and improve their own care.

What Do We Mean by the Right Care?

Jane's Story

I had cervical cancer, diagnosed early thank God, but my gynaecologist wanted to remove my whole womb to have the best chance of a cure. I wanted just the cancer removed and to keep my womb to give me the best chance of having a baby. We had a long conversation, I took my time to decide and he didn't pressure me but he made it clear that his main focus was to do everything possible to stop the cancer returning. I chose my way, my gorgeous baby is now eighteen years old and I have learned to live with the chance of the cancer returning. Other women I know have not been so lucky.

Mica's Story

Four years ago our daughter had brain cancer – a medulloblastoma, the same one as Ashya King – and had surgery to remove it. Her oncologist wanted her to have radiotherapy because she believed it offers the best chance of cure, but we – like the Kings – wanted to consider a newer radiation treatment, proton beam therapy, because there might be less chance of side effects. The NHS protocol for radiotherapy had four pages on side effects – on brain function, academic ability, fertility, growth, hearing, cataracts, the possibility of sowing the seeds for future cancers. That seemed a heavy price for survival. Medicine is founded on 'first do no harm', or failing that, 'do least harm'.

We researched proton beam therapy and there was less evidence to back it up but it did seem to cause less damage to normal tissue and we spoke to parents who said the side effects of radiotherapy were long term, but they are less than they used to be because the technology is better. We talked it through a lot. Our oncologist said she didn't think our choice was the best from a 'trying to stop the cancer returning' point of view but understood it might be the best from our 'do less harm' point of view. Proton beam therapy wasn't available in the NHS – and still isn't – but the NHS will fund it if your oncologist and a funding panel agree. We would have to be in America for ten weeks and go as quickly as possible, because the sooner treatment started the better. It was a very difficult and stressful time for us as my mother was very ill as well and in the end we stayed and had radiotherapy in the NHS. Our daughter came through the treatment but it was unpleasant and she does have side effects – particularly concentration, thinking and memory – and we'll never truly know how much it has affected her, or how she would have been after PBT. When I read about Ashya King, it makes me wonder whether I did the best for my daughter, which is hard to take. My husband is more pragmatic. He said we made the best decision for us at the time, but the instinct for a mother to protect her child from harm – and the guilt you feel if you think you haven't done your best – is lifelong.

Raj's Story

I needed a hip replacement and my surgeon recommended a brand new metal-on-metal hip. I asked him what the alternatives were but he said this one was the best and newest, and was much less likely to wear out, whatever I did. I didn't fancy something new that hadn't been used in humans before, so I asked for another opinion – which wasn't that easy to get and I had to wait. But I'm so glad I did. The second surgeon recommended a very old-fashioned Exeter hip. He said I shouldn't go anywhere near a metal-on-metal hip. He said the potential risks were far too high and I didn't need to take them at my age. He said I needed a tried-and-tested hip with great results that was just right for a man of sixty-eight. My new hip works a treat and I was so relieved when I read about all the metal hips that have failed. How can two surgeons a few miles apart give you such different opinions?

As these three stories illustrate, healthcare choices are far from easy, and what's right for one person, or what a doctor thinks is right for you, may not be what you think is right for you. Modern medicine has considerable power to harm as well as to help. New isn't always better, and more isn't always better. Too much diagnosis, testing and treatment can do more harm than good, as happy people are turned into anxious patients.

The flip side of scepticism in a publicly-funded system that demands more evidence before paying for treatments is that the NHS does not always offer drugs or new technologies available in the rest of Europe, delays their introduction or restricts their use more tightly. In a private system, the customer has more freedom to choose what risks he or she is prepared to take, and there is a danger of being oversold something of dubious or limited benefit when you're ill and desperate. But if a treatment turns out to be a real breakthrough, some NHS patients who would have benefited from early introduction miss out.

A further problem is that proper scientific trials are difficult and expensive, and decisions often have to be made on the basis of imperfect or incomplete evidence. Even if a treatment offers some proven benefit the NHS may reject it as too expensive. Yet despite the apparently cautious approach of the NHS, thousands of new metal-on-metal hip replacements were recently used in NHS centres (and across the world) when there were safer, proven alternatives, because some surgeons and patients swallowed the marketing hype and didn't take time to properly weigh up the risks and benefits. Many of these hip replacements have now failed, caused a huge amount of damage requiring removal and repeat surgery, and mass legal action has followed which the NHS and the manufacturers will have to share the cost for.

To repeat, only you can decide how involved you want to be in decisions about your care, but the evidence suggests that the more involved you are, and are allowed to be, the more likely you are to get the right care for you. Only you can decide – having considered the risks – if your wish to have a child is more important than minimizing your risk of a cancer returning. Or whether you want to fight for a less-proven radiation therapy for your child's brain if it might cause fewer long-term side effects. As patients and parents are encouraged to take on more responsibility for difficult choices, the NHS has to adapt to let you in.

effective. You won't be able to have much say in how your hip replacement is put in at the time, but you can ask about the process. If you want to know what the process of, say, your asthma care should be, then the NICE website will tell you what care you should be getting (e.g. have you got an asthma plan that tells you what to do if your illness deteriorates?). Knowing the description and standards of care you should be getting puts you in a better position to speak up if you're not getting it.

4) Experience

If your experience of care has been good, it's more likely that the end result (outcome) will be good too. Again, NICE has defined what the experience of every patient using the NHS should be and it's worth reading and reflecting on whether yours matches up to this (see later). By sharing your experience on public websites you can guide other patients, and you can also use these websites to find services in the NHS which patients rate very highly (e.g. iWantGreatCare). Sharing your experience also lets patients know what to expect (e.g. healthtalk. org) and helps the NHS to improve and address any immediate problems you have (e.g. Patient Opinion).

5) Outcome

It's not always easy to judge the end result of your care, particularly if most of it is about preventing illness rather than treating it. The overall aim of the NHS is to improve your life by giving you the care that's right for you, but in a messy, chaotic system this care will sometimes veer off track. However, you can help get it back on track if you have access to your data and medical records, and you've learned about the treatment you've opted for, and what the process, experience and outcome should be.

You might also look at the NHS outcome data and ask to be referred to an NHS service that has a lot of expertise in managing your condition, gets good results and has a good safety record. The new My NHS or My Cancer Treatment websites are promising to give you this data, but it's too early to say how accurate and useful it will be, or how many patients will opt to use it. League tables of results may be flawed if they don't take fairly take into account say, surgeons who do harder operations on sicker patients, or hospitals that serve poorer and sicker populations. And they may even discourage some doctors from taking on the sickest patients. But the NHS is about to release more public data than any health service in the world, and also to give you secure access to your own health records. If it gets it right, this drive towards transparency and openness is to be welcomed. You don't have to look at any of it, but it's there if you want to.

All health and social care services in England, both private and NHS, are inspected, regulated and rated by the Care Quality Commission (CQC). In theory, you can use this information to guide where you choose to be treated and cared for – GP practices, dentists, care homes and hospitals. And if you come across care that is unacceptable, you should also tell the CQC. As patients and carers, you are the smoke alarms for poor care and are usually the first to pick up problems.

Raising the Bar on Your NHS Care

The best care you can get from the NHS is not always the best that modern medicine has to offer, it's *the best care possible in the circumstances*. No country can afford the highest standards of care for all its citizens at all times, and half of all doctors and hospitals will always be below average for any particular treatment. If you get suddenly sick, you have no control over when it happens, where you are taken or what the queues are like ahead of you. The right care needs the right diagnosis but it can also depend on you getting the right information at the right time and choosing a treatment that is right for you, and then doing your best to help it succeed. Health decisions will not always be right first time, but there is always something you and your carers can do to raise the bar on your care. And to do that, you need to think of the NHS as a partnership, rather than a service.

You won't always get brilliant 'highest-bar' care when you use the NHS, but your care should always clear the lower-level 'safety' bar. This is the minimum standard of cleanliness, kindness, competence and safety that should happen for all NHS care. It won't always happen in an overloaded system, which is why it's important to speak up if you spot something that doesn't appear clean, kind, competent or safe. You have to think of yourself as an active partner in your care, not a passive recipient. The upper bar is for high-quality care where you share decisions about what is best for you, and this care is delivered to the highest standards possible with you participating as much as you can to help it succeed. This is the quality of care the NHS aspires to but needs your help to reach.

A good mind-set when using the NHS is to hope for the best (high-quality care), prepare for the most likely (in-between the quality and safety bars) and have an emergency plan for the worst (below the safety bar). Some NHS care clears the high-quality bar, most is somewhere between the two bars and some falls short of the safety bar. If you have to use the NHS a lot, you'll find that the level of the bar can vary a lot from place to place, and time to time. There are different strategies, and different levels of urgency, for these different situations, but your daily goal should always be to try to raise the bar on your care, little by little, so you're always above the safety bar, joining in and joining up your care and living a life of joy, hope, purpose and meaning within the limits of your illness. When your time comes, you also deserve the best death possible – and that takes thought and planning too.

A better title for this book could be how to get the best *with* the NHS. It takes knowledge, skills, courage and energy to turn the NHS from a spectator sport to a true partnership between patients, carers and staff. To inspire you, this book has plenty of examples of those who've got more involved, taken on more control and responsibility, raised the bar on their care and lived better lives as a result. None of this is easy when you're ill, but most NHS care is about improving the lives of those with long-term conditions that aren't going away in a hurry. Many people are now living with these diseases for fifty years or more. Once you get over the shock of the diagnosis, you realize that for 99 per cent of your time, you're the one treating yourself and controlling your care. The NHS is just an extension of your self-care, and you should continue to treat yourself and control your care as much as you can when you use it.

There will clearly be times when you are too confused, distressed, fatigued or frail to be an active participant in your care. Your carers then become your advocates, and need to be involved in your care as much as you want them to be. Again, this is more likely to happen if you're able to think and plan in advance. Occasionally the system breaks down and either offers dangerous and disjointed care, no access to care or even unkind care. There are few things harder in life than tackling an illness and the failings in the NHS and social care system, but humans are remarkably resilient when they have to be. One of the keys to getting better healthcare is to be as emotionally healthy as you can be outside the NHS, and to take your knowledge, skills, interests and values into it. Your care can only be personalized if the people treating you know you as a person.

There are countless ways that you could raise the bar, and not all of them will ring bells with you. Time may be limited, but the things you could do with that time are almost limitless. Don't waste it obsessing about your health or the health service, but make sure when you do have to use it that you go in with your eyes open.

The Right Team

The NHS is a very complex organization employing 1.5 million people across the UK, and there are hundreds of different people and professionals you could encounter (and careers you could potentially apply for – see www.nhscareers.nhs.uk). Unless you ask, you won't always be told the name of the person treating you, let alone their qualifications, what they're intending to do to you, why and how it fits in with your overall treatment plan. The NHS is getting better at communication and teamwork, but it's still not that unusual for patients to be unaware of what medication they're taking and why, or what has happened to them (even when they've had surgery). It's just as likely that different members of the large team treating you won't have communicated and shared vital information, increasing the chance that you might get the wrong care, suboptimal care or unnecessary repetition of investigations.

To get great care, you need to know who's caring for you. If you don't know who someone is, and they don't tell you, ask. Here's one of my favourite patient stories from Ralph, aged sixty-seven.

'WHO ARE YOU? AND WHAT ARE YOUR GOALS FOR ME TODAY?'

Ralph's Story

When you've been a patient for a while, you learn how to take some control. When I'm in hospital, I have a big card at the head of my bed that says:

Who are you?

What is your job?

What are you planning to do with me?

Why?

Now wash your hands.

Anyone who comes near me gets asked those questions or, if I'm tired, I point to the card. I won't let anyone touch me if I don't know their name, their qualifications, their intended actions and their reasons why. And I don't always agree. Some staff are a bit terse, but most of them are fine. Especially when they realize what I went through with MRSA. And now they know me, the good ones do it graciously without me having to ask. But I'm always surprised by the number of NHS staff who are clueless when you ask them, 'What are your goals for me today?' All teams must have goals, and my goals are written on the other side of the card. Everyone in the team has to read them and discuss them with me. Then they have to wash their hands. Otherwise, they're not in my team. I'd advise every patient to do the same. It's quite easy to get the hang of 'Who? What? What? Why? Wash!' Especially when it's written on a card on your bed.

Ralph is delightful company when he's away from the NHS (I met him at a patient safety conference, where he told me about the devastating impact of his hospital-acquired infection). Inside the NHS, I'm guessing he's also delightful company and an active partner in his care with those who've earned his trust. But if he isn't sure about what's happening, he speaks up assertively. Good teamwork allows people to disagree and challenge each other in a respectful way. Raising the bar on your care is often hard work, and a joint effort. But it's much easier if you know and understand who's in your team, and you all try to work in one joined-up system with clear goals that you've all under-stood and agreed to.

Who Is in Your Team?

For any serious illness, there will be a lot of people involved in your care. As well as knowing the standards of care you should be getting, you also need to make your own map of crucial team members, who they are and how to contact them. If your treatment is complicated, you may see lots of different specialists and other NHS staff in different buildings who don't always communicate. You need a navigator to write out a map of who is who, and what they do.

For example, if you have bowel cancer, you might at some stage be cared for by:

- GPs, nurses, healthcare assistants and the primary care team

- Colorectal surgeons

- Radiation oncologists

- Medical oncologists

- Radiologists

- Urologists

- Gastroenterologists

- Pain specialists

- Stoma therapists

- Interventional radiologists

- Neurosurgeons

- Anaesthetists

- Dieticians

- Psychologists

- Radiographers

- Pharmacists

- Healthcare assistants

- Physiotherapists

- Occupational therapists

- Operating department practitioners

- Nurse practitioners

- Nurse consultants

- Physician assistants

- Social workers

- Genetic counsellors

- Paramedics

- Macmillan nurses

- The hospice and palliative care team

That's a huge team to try to get your head around when you're ill, and there are plenty of other professionals and people who work as part of the wider NHS and social care team that try to keep the show on the road. You also want to include yourself, and your carers as part of the team, and it may be that it's a healthcare assistant, porter, chaplain, receptionist, ward clerk, cleaner, volunteer or student who is the most important person to you. Kindness and support in the NHS often comes most from those who are paid the least, in training or giving their time for free.

A single person linking all these other people together for you makes a huge difference. The NHS is currently considering the role of an 'NHS and social care navigator' who may end up being one of the most important people to patients, your 'go to' person who glues it all together and takes a huge amount of pressure off yourself and your carers.

In the meantime, charities are always extremely helpful in explaining the care you should be getting, and who in the NHS does what (e.g. www.bowelcanceruk.org.uk). And using the experiences of others can be very helpful in knowing what to expect and seeking out the right care for you. The healthtalk.org website is a great starting point. Try to get to know your team as people, thank them but don't be shy to raise concerns and put them to the test when you need to. If you don't have a navigator, ask who your 'go to' person is at each step on the journey (e.g. it could be a named GP, district nurse or specialist cancer nurse at any stage).

Trackers: Another Checklist for the Right NHS Care

Checklists are great for cutting through the anxiety, chaos and hierarchy in the NHS and reminding you what matters to you now. If you're having surgery, check out the Surgical Safety checklist and ask to be included when they go through it before your operation. Checklists work best if you make your own or personalize someone else's. What's important for me may not be as important for you. The checklist I use when I'm analysing patient's stories as a journalist and a doctor is TRACKERS. It may help you pinpoint the problem in your care and get your care back on track if it goes off.

The Right Care is . . .

> **T**ransparent
> **R**ight for You
> **A**ccessible and **A**ccountable
> **C**ompetent and **C**ollaborative
> **K**ind
> **E**ffective
> **R**ight first time
> **S**afe

TRANSPARENT . . . You have all the information you need about your illness, your medical records, treatment options and the safety, quality, standards and results of the team treating you – and how they compare with other NHS units.

RIGHT for you . . . There is usually more than one treatment option and sharing that decision, understanding the risks and benefits and agreeing what's best for you is more likely to be successful than just going with a doctor's opinion. Most decisions don't need to be rushed. So take your time.

ACCESSIBLE and **ACCOUNTABLE . . .** Choosing the right care is no good if you can't get access to it within a reasonable time (the *NHS Handbook* tells you what the maximum waiting time should be). You also need easy access to your medical records, data and support. Simple text support on a mobile phone can make a huge difference. For any treatment, you need the name of someone – e.g. a senior doctor or nurse – who is ultimately accountable for your care, who agrees goals with you and is your 'go to' person for serious concerns.

COMPETENT and **COLLABORATIVE . . .** Treatment should be agreed to standards by properly trained staff on safely staffed wards. Working together as a team, and joining up and sharing information with other NHS and social care teams is the best route to great care, but often you have to do a lot of the joining up yourself to stop falling through the cracks in the NHS and social care system.

KIND . . . Healthcare without kindness is pointless, rotten and inexcusable. Just because we *can* do something doesn't mean we *should.* Always consider – is more treatment less humane? And are the basic needs of food, water, communication, pain relief and toileting being met?

EFFECTIVE . . . You are the best judge of whether your treatment has made a positive difference to your life in the long term, and you should feed this information back so the NHS learns to improve and knows what, and what not, to spend public money on.

RIGHT first time . . . This won't always happen, but it is more likely to happen if you understand what should be happening to you, and the standard of care you should be getting. Even so, you will not always go seamlessly from the right diagnosis to the right treatment, and errors and bad luck can and will occur at any stage. If treatment that should be working isn't working, go right back to the start. Is the diagnosis right? What else could it be? Have I been given the right treatment in the right way? Or was I just unlucky?

SAFE . . . Patients and carers can sense how safe the NHS is within a few minutes of stepping on to a ward or into a surgery. If it looks chaotic, understaffed and overstretched, it almost certainly is. Missing or delaying vital drugs to stop infection and blood clots are common causes of harm, as are failures to spot serious deteriorations in a patient's condition quickly. That's when you as carers need to step up, ask what you can do to help and keep your eyes open on your loved one and the competence and cleanliness of the team treating him or her. You don't have to make a diagnosis, but you can tell when a person or room is dirty, and you may spot your mum getting rapidly sicker and needing urgent attention. Often patients and carers spot a problem before the staff. You are the smoke alarm for NHS harm. But you have to be heard.

THE RIGHT INFORMATION AND SUPPORT AT THE RIGHT TIME

Information can give you both power and freedom in all walks of life, but it needs to be accurate and you may need support to understand or come to terms with it. Information that has been factually verified is called knowledge, and it can be as powerful as any medicine. And like a drug, it has to be used wisely. As the humorist Miles Kington put it: 'Knowledge is knowing a tomato is a fruit. Wisdom is knowing not to put one in a fruit salad.' The context in which knowledge is used is as important as the knowledge itself.

Dr Muir Gray, one of my NHS heroes, likens knowledge to water. Patients and NHS staff need it instantly and on tap, but it has to be pure, and not contaminated with bad science, bias and vested interest. If you have the skills, you can learn to read a newspaper story or analyse a scientific paper and spot the limitations and bias (the *NHS Behind the Headlines* site is a good place to start). But most of us just want the pure knowledge on tap without having to do the difficult analysis. The knowledge you get from reliable websites should be free from bias but some human errors are inevitable.

Knowledge from research is called evidence. The NHS aims only to offer treatments that are evidence-based, i.e. that have been proven to work in clinical trials, with the added restriction that NICE must have judged them to offer good value for money to the NHS as well. In reality, the NHS still offers lots of screening and treatment that doesn't have a very solid evidence base, and for some – particularly rare – conditions the evidence is lacking and so a certain amount of guesswork based on experience is needed. And no-one really knows the true benefits and harms of older patients taking so many different drugs at the same time.

Knowledge from healthcare performance is called statistics. There is a limit, in any health service, as to how much benefit you get back from the money you put in. Increasing the funding of the health service twenty-fold over the years has coincided with a steady rise in life expectancy but it certainly hasn't made us twenty times healthier. Putting money into education and giving all children the knowledge, skills, confidence and courage to get better jobs and make better decisions about their health might achieve more than very expensive, high-tech healthcare.

Knowledge can also be particular to you and the service you are using. If you want to, you can learn about your medical records, the performance of the team and organization treating you, what other patients and NHS staff think of their care and whether their life improved as a result of it. This focus on outcomes has to be set in context (poorer areas have more disease and lower life expectancies because of it, so blaming the NHS for this is unfair). But more information is now available than ever before for patients who want to research and seek the best care possible – or choose none at all. If patients are given more information, you don't tend to use more healthcare, you use less.

When you're ill, you can move from self-care, to informal care from family and voluntary help, to generalist NHS care, to social care, to specialist and even super-specialist care. But wherever you are on that journey, you need the right information and support at the right time. We have to use this information to break down the barriers between these different levels of care. We have to work more like an ant colony to get the best from the NHS. Neither markets nor more bureaucracy can solve the challenges facing the NHS. Giving patients the knowledge to get the right care and be free from the wrong care or unnecessary over-treatment is the key.

Remember, all healthcare should have a process (a clearly defined way of doing something according to agreed standards) and an outcome (the end result). The outcome is crucially dependent on the process (to get the right results, you need to do the right things right) but sometimes you can get compassionate care delivered to the best standards but it just doesn't get the results you hoped for. There is always an element of luck involved.

. You can influence the process and outcome of your care by checking your diagnosis, chasing your results and referral, choosing the treatment you think is best for you, choosing the team you think is best placed to deliver it, finding out about your illness, treatment, rights and standards and checking that they're being followed, and doing whatever you can to stick to the plan and recover. You may be too frail, confused or exhausted to do anything other than let the experts get on with it. Or you may prefer to wing it and put all your energy into building good relationships with the staff. The amount you want to get involved may vary from day to day. But it's crucial that if you want to be more involved in your care, you let everybody know. You may have to speak up to get your place at the table. And wise up to be fully involved in decisions about your care.

Processes in the NHS are often idealized, rather than real. They tell you what care you should be getting, but not what to do of you don't get it. The NHS Constitution gives you a map of the NHS as a whole – its principles and values, and your rights and responsibilities. But you also need larger-scale maps for specific circumstances. 'The Map of Medicine', available through the NHS website, is a great invention that shows you quickly and succinctly the various steps in the journey from diagnosis to treatment for a wide range of conditions. The wonderful healthtalk.org website is full of real stories from patients and carers to let you know what the various steps on that journey felt like to them, and what you can expect from your experiences. And NICE defines quality standards – maps based on the best evidence to guide you through the care you should be getting, and prompting you to ask questions when you're not.

NICE, like the rest of the NHS, is not immune to error and vested interest, and needs to be scrutinized. Many of the experts who sit on panels to decide, say, whether statins should be given to lower the cholesterol of lower-risk patients, have links with the drug companies that make them. Even if these links are openly declared, some people believe the guidance may be biased towards over-treatment.

You won't always get the best care medicine can offer in the NHS, but you should have a say in where the bar is set for your care, and also what level of care you're prepared to accept when you can't get the best. If you don't speak up about something that concerns you, that concern may well not be addressed. NHS staff are generally kind and hardworking, but we're not clairvoyants.

Patients who have a good experience of NHS care are more likely to get better results from their care. Success can never be guaranteed, but unkind care is always harmful. So the NICE quality standard for patient experience is important to help judge whether your experience of NHS care is up to the highest standard. It's made up of fourteen statements that describe high-quality care for patients, which NICE says is 'the best care you should receive'. When you're giving feedback, either to praise excellent care or raise concerns about aspects of your care, it has a lot more clout if you can reference it to the specific standard statements you think are not being met.

According to NICE, as an NHS patient you *should* . . .

1. Be treated with dignity, kindness, compassion, courtesy, respect, understanding and honesty.

2. Be cared for by staff who can communicate with you in a clear and understandable way.

3. Be introduced to all healthcare professionals involved in your care, and made aware of the roles and responsibilities of the members of the healthcare team.

4. Have opportunities to discuss your health beliefs, concerns and preferences, and have these taken into account when making decisions about your care.

5. Be helped by healthcare professionals to understand relevant treatment options, including benefits, risks and potential consequences of care.

6. Be actively involved in making decisions about your care, and supported to make fully informed choices about investigations, treatment and care that reflect what is important to you.

7. Have your choices respected and supported when deciding whether to accept or decline treatment, and when choosing between treatments.

8. Be made aware that you can ask for a second opinion.

9. Experience care that is tailored to your needs and personal preferences, taking into account your circumstances, how easy it is for you to use the services you need, and any other health problems you have.

10. Be regularly checked and asked whether you need any extra support, for example with eating and drinking, pain relief, continence problems or anxieties.

11. See the same healthcare professional or healthcare team throughout a course of treatment whenever this is possible.

12. Expect information about your care to be exchanged in a clear and accurate way between relevant health and social care professionals, so that your care is coordinated with the least possible delay or disruption.

13. Be asked if you want your partner, family members and/or carers to be given information about your care, and have your preferences respected and reviewed throughout your care.

14. Be given clear advice about who to contact about your healthcare needs, how to contact you and when to contact you.

Take a moment to consider the last time you, a friend or relative used the NHS. How many of the standards were met? Did the missing ones matter? Did it affect the quality of your care? How much effort were you able to put into participating and raising the standards in your care? Did it make a difference?

Like the declaration of your rights in the NHS Constitution, this NICE standard is useful as a checklist not just during a hospital stay, but to make sure you've covered all the bases before discharge home from hospital. It also applies to care in general practice and in other community services. It should make it easier for you and your carers to be involved as a team – you should have a named person in charge of your care and details of how to contact him or her. Basic but fundamental needs such as eating, drinking, pain relief and toileting should be regularly checked. Important doses of medications such as antibiotics and clot-preventing drugs should not be delayed or missed. Sometimes, the NHS is so crowded, you may have to chase after your care, check blood results are back, and record and share important information with different members of the team. Don't be shy about being a chaser. Better healthcare is more likely to be right first time with fewer errors and less repetition. It usually costs the NHS less and helps other patients, rather than leapfrogs over them.

Technology is key to getting information and support to you when you need it, delivered at the right time in the right way, so you can take control over your care. Here's one of my favourite examples.

'IT'S A LOT EASIER HAVING A NURSE IN YOUR POCKET.'

Josh's Story

Josh has diabetes that he struggles to cope with and control, and had forty-six hospital admissions in one year. He was asked if he wanted to use Flo, a simple system that uses his own mobile phone (or landline) to communicate with NHS staff. It's web-based, so doctors and nurses can access Flo anywhere and immediately put the patient on whatever protocol is most clinically appropriate. Josh's diabetes is so hard to control, he gives readings five times a day rather than the usual three.

'I felt like I lost my independence with the diabetes, I had to rely on a lot of other people. And I had denial issues so I had to rely on my Nan, and my parents had to kick me up the backside to try to make me do the tests but still I was in denial. I'd rather just not do it at the time. I just hated it and I needed to take control. I think the worst thing is emotionally, seeing your parents upset about it all, and you realize you have to get yourself out of it. It's still hard, even today I still struggle with it, I'm not going to lie. But it's a lot easier than it was. I was going into hospital five times a month, now it's once or twice every three or four months. So it's gone down massively and it's a lot easier to control.

'It's a lot easier having your own on-hand "nurse". I was having a routine appointment, just like a chat because me and my nurse get on very well. She knows my story quite well, so we spoke about it and she said there's a new idea coming along called Flo, would I be interested in trying it, and I was just at my lowest, I was ready to try anything. Out of everything I've tried over the years, it turned out to be the simplest, the easiest and the best option out of the lot. It's actually an easy system to use because it's on hand, so you don't have to rely on calling the surgery, you don't have to wait for hours on end for appointments, and it's the same with any medication if you need that little prompt or that little nag to take it, it's right there giving you a message. I get five messages a day that prompt me to test my blood sugars, it gives me good advice, it gives me good replies, and the reply time is absolutely fantastic, it's under a minute and I get a reply with knowing what to do if I have a problem.

'There are still hospital visits, but it's nowhere near as gargantuan as it was before and it makes it so much easier to have that little on-hand nurse in your pocket to give you those constant little prompts. Setting it up was really quick and easy – within the first day of even mentioning it, I had an appointment within a week to see my trainer, within a few hours all my details were on the system and by the end of the day I was getting my first messages and I started switching my life around. It took under a few hours to sort everything out. I recommend it should be rolled out absolutely everywhere. If it can help me come out the dumps, it can help anyone. I was in a really, really bad place, not just with health, but emotional wise, I was very lucky I didn't have to go on antidepressants and I managed to control it with determination to get through it. And Flo helped me do it.'

Flo is a very simple system just about anyone can use to manage and monitor a whole range of diseases via their phone. Buddy is a similar system for psychological support and treatment monitoring. If you want to try either, ask your GP and nurse if they can set it, or a similar scheme, up for you.

It's impossible for you to participate fully in your NHS care if you aren't given all your information and data. If you have a complicated history and are having to see lots of doctors who don't know you, make sure you know your medical story, drugs, investigations and diagnosis. You are allowed to see and copy your medical records (www. nhs.uk tells you how), and you should gather copies of all the letters written about you as they go to and from hospital or community clinics. Think 'nothing about me, without me'. The more you know about your care, the more likely you can keep it on track and stop mistakes. If your notes are complex, take a summary along with you whenever you use the NHS.

Some practices give you easy access to your medical records online. Your GP's website could be as good as the one set up by GP Dr Amir Hannan at www.htmc.co.uk. Dr Hannan is another one of my NHS heroes. He responded to the challenge of taking over the medical practice of the mass murderer Dr Harold Shipman, who killed at least 250 patients, by making his GP practice one of the most honest, open, transparent and technologically savvy in the UK. Dr Hannan realized that he had to re-establish trust, and one way to do that was to encourage as many patients who wanted it to have complete access to their medical records. Anything written about them, they could plainly see. They could be fully involved in all decisions about their care. Nothing about you, without you.

He started out by offering all patients a copy of their records on a USB stick that they could carry around with them. Now he offers them the same service online. Over the years, Dr Hannan has built up this culture of transparency, and patients in his practice participate not just in decisions about their own care but in the running of the practice and its continual improvement. The technology has been important not in itself, but because it's driven this culture change where patients are given all their personal medical information and data if they wish it, they can book appointments and order prescriptions online, update information to and correct their own records and they can take on as much responsibility for their care as they want to. There is no reason why your GP practice shouldn't be able to offer this service, and they may already be. Many patients miss out on better care simply by not realizing it exists. You don't know what you don't know. So ask to have access to your data and keep and carry copies of vital information (dates, doctors, diagnoses, tests, treatments, all letters written about you, drug names and doses, what they're for, who started them, how and for how long you should take them). You don't have to remember this all in your head (not even doctors can do that) but you need to have easy access to all this information because different parts of the NHS often won't. The right information at the right time can be a life-saver.

New technology to give patients more control over their care works best when doctors are equally enthusiastic about handing over control. One great system, called Patients Know Best, allows NHS teams and patients to work as true partners through a secure 'Facebook-style' website where patients can access their records at any time, organize them in a way they can understand, add to them, upload 'traffic light' monitoring systems and advice that tells them what to do if an illness gets worse, and to share their records (or not share them) with anyone they choose. This allows online conversations, and Skype, with many members of a team and family at once. Some hospitals and GP practices use their own computer systems to allow you access to your notes online, but Patients Know Best (PKB) is the most interactive system I've come across, giving you control, not just access. It requires your NHS team to upload your records and work with you, so you need to ask them if they're using the system, or something similar. However, it's leading the way in the NHS to a move towards more online consulting and less taking a day out of your life to drive to, park and hang around a hospital or surgery.

This system is very good for patients with chronic diseases – asthma, diabetes and those with inflammatory bowel disease – where you have to manage your own condition every day of your life. To do it as well as you can, you should have as much control over your data and information as you want to have. You need moral support too, but with PKB you can involve the whole team. You can upload absolutely anything to your secure website, all your consultant letters, research you've done, etc, automatically. You can even add your end of life choices. The traffic light protocols for what action to take if your symptoms get worse are brilliant. You know exactly what to do if your condition deteriorates, how to seek help, scale up your treatment and prevent hospital admission wherever possible. There is even a PKB app for the phone and whenever you contact PKB you get a quick reply. If you're a bit worried about a blood result you can get a quick answer, rather than stew over it all weekend. You can also upload all your records onto your phone for travel. You can keep a copy downloaded if you don't have access to wireless so wherever you go in the world, if you fall ill the medical staff will know all about you and your disease quickly. It gives people the confidence to travel and enjoy life and live well with illness.

Patients Know Best has been taken up more by specialist units in hospitals so far than in general practice, but the potential is there for one key health-carer (e.g. Mum) to have access to and control over the whole family's medical records and hence oversee all their care, check what drugs need renewing, what immunizations have been given, when others are due, what the asthma management plan is, etc. It's extraordinary what people can do for themselves with the right training and support, and a fair dollop of courage and encouragement. But the right care always needs the right information at the right time.

If you're the kind of person who likes monitoring your data, there are all sorts of apps available on the NHS and Patient.co.uk website to track your health, fitness and any chronic diseases you may have (depression, diabetes, heart disease, lung disease). Before choosing, see what if any trials have been done to show that they improve care. Most health apps barely get used, so ask the team treating you which they recommend and which are compatible with their computer system so you can share data easily. Apple has just launched health-monitoring apps to link up with the NHS computer system EMIS (which your GP may or may not use). Some people like to feel on top of their diseases and data, others dislike the intrusion into their lives. If a disease needs close monitoring to motivate you and keep you well, apps can be very helpful. Some are being developed to feed back automatically to your medical records and GP practice (with your consent – you're the one who should keep control of your own data, and how it's used).

THE RIGHT SELF-CARE

We are very good at caring for ourselves, and the human body is remarkably good at healing itself given the time. Seventy-five per cent of us have some sort of symptom every fortnight, but only 8 per cent of us see a GP. We sort out 90 per cent of our symptoms without coming anywhere near the NHS and when we do, 90 per cent of problems are sorted out by GP care (for only 8 per cent of the budget). There are lots of good sources of help and information you can try that are often easier than seeing a GP and much less hassle for you. Most of the information leaflets your GP or nurse gives you are freely available at www. patient.co.uk and www.nhs.uk and both of these websites have 'symptom sorters' to guide you to the most likely diagnosis, whether it's likely to get better on its own, how long you should wait and see, and any red flags that suggest you need an urgent appointment. Dr Hannan's website – www.htmc.co.uk – is also a great and easy source of information, linking up to other great health websites.

The NHS 'Choose Well' advice is excellent, although they've stopped printing the leaflets so you may have to get it online. Your local NHS should personalize the information, for example Manchester's www. choosewellmanchester.org.uk is a truly excellent site. Patient.co.uk has excellent information, apps, advice and videos from the outstanding GP, Dr Sarah Jarvis. Also, www.selfcareforum.org tells you how to care for yourself, how long you should leave symptoms before seeking help, and what 'red flag' symptoms trump all the other advice and tell you to get help. Fifty-two million GP consultations a year are still for conditions that get better on their own, and around fifty million people can't get consultations with their GPs when they want to – some of whom really need them. So if you can get help elsewhere, you could free up a consultation for someone who really needs it.

Most ailments (coughs, colds, earaches, skin rashes, muscular aches and sprains) get better in time, even without treatment. But you do have to be patient. For example:

- Ninety per cent of coughs last up to three weeks and will not be helped by antibiotics unless you are elderly, very ill or have another health condition.

- Ear infections (acute otitis media) are usually over in four days.

- Sore throats take a week to heal.

- The common cold can take ten days to recover from.

- Sinus infections take up to two and a half weeks to clear.

None of these needs antibiotics unless you, or your child, develops complications. And the above websites have lots of information on spotting complications. Often you won't need any drugs for minor ailments. They just get better in time. Supermarkets are allowed to sell drugs off the shelf that are on the General Sales List (e.g. painkillers) and your pharmacist can give you all sorts of expert advice on a wide range of conditions, and sell you a lot of stronger 'P list' medications after a consultation to check they're right for you. Antibiotic drops for conjunctivitis, emergency contraception, all sorts of thrush treatments and strong drugs to stop stomach acid are all available without the need for a prescription. If you get your prescriptions free and don't want to pay, your pharmacist may run a minor ailment scheme, that gives you a consultation and a free prescription that your GP signs off later. Ask.

If you prefer getting your information from a book rather than a website, *Diagnosing Your Health Symptoms for Dummies* by GP Dr Knut Schroeder is a great book to have in your house (or on your iPad). It gives excellent information about when and how to care for yourself, and when to seek NHS help – although this information is widely available for free on the above websites. Your own GP knows your past medical history and has access to your medical records (as you should) and can provide extra advice and reassurance, but in most cases it won't be needed. If you find the right information on these reliable websites, test and talk through your decision to care for yourself with friends and family, you'll discover the vast majority of symptoms get better if you give yourself time to heal, without needing any NHS intervention. However, it does often take time.

THE RIGHT EMERGENCY CARE

In an emergency situation, you don't have the luxury of time. Getting the right emergency care in the NHS is crucially dependent on you spotting the emergency, calling for urgent help and giving what life support you can.

In an emergency when someone has collapsed, been poisoned, is contemplating or has attempted suicide, lost consciousness, has chest pain, breathing difficulties or sudden loss of blood, movement, sensation, speech or vision – then don't waste time calling your GP or 111 – call 999. The possible exception is in very isolated communities where some GPs are emergency responders. Paramedics are generally well trained to deal with emergencies and you need to get to a specialist hospital unit fast. It's worth knowing where your nearest specialist units are for heart attacks and strokes to ensure your friend or relative is being taken there. It's also worth knowing what their end of life wishes are, and whether they want emergency treatment.

If you phone 999, the person assessing the call may not classify it as urgent. The more knowledge, information and life-support training you have, the more able you are to give an accurate description of the urgency. Reading around the subject on the NHS and Patient.co.uk websites can help, and they also provide information about how and when to phone 999, and what to do before help arrives. There are also some great apps (e.g. from St John Ambulance) you can download on your phone. But there is no substitute for learning basic life support skills and keeping them up to date. You never know when you may need them.

'SHE DIDN'T CRY OR SHOUT FOR HELP, SHE JUST STARTED TURNING BLUE'

Grant's Story

I've done some first aid training at work but you never actually think you're going to need it. Medical emergencies are what happen to other people. We were sitting down to our Sunday lunch and it was quite a busy table. The kids enjoy their food but they also enjoy talking and I try to tell them not to talk and eat at the same time. Often they don't take any notice and I don't push it.

My youngest daughter was sitting opposite me at the far end of the table. She is five and she likes her food and the sound of her own voice and so do I, but for me food always trumps conversation. Normally I get in the zone when there's a plateful of food in front of me and it's quite hard to distract me. So I don't know what made me look up and look at Lucy. Oddly, I think it may be because she was quieter than normal. All the other kids were chattering away and ignoring her and she just went silent. I think I even heard a little slurp of a bit of meat getting sucked down into her airway. She didn't cry or shout for help she just started turning blue and nobody else spotted it. I didn't really have time to think about it. I think having done the drills before helped but it still felt like I was moving in slow motion. I just grabbed her, put her over my knees with her head down and did some back blows. And a bit of beef came flying out.

I can remember choking as a child on a boiled sweet, and my dad just picked me up by my legs, hung me upside down and out it came. But I was making a hell of a racket trying to cough it out. I never realized you could choke silently, but I do now. And I've learned to notice stuff and trust my instincts, particularly with the

children's health. And now we never talk when we have a mouthful,
but we do in between mouthfuls and it's made me slow down my
eating and enjoy meal times more.

Anyone can learn life support skills, and everyone should from an
early age. If you collapsed, would your children know how to dial
999? Emergencies such as heart attacks and strokes have their seeds
sown silently over many years but then strike very quickly, often
with severe symptoms that you haven't had before of pain, nausea or
just feeling awful. There may be someone nearby who remembers
the Vinnie Jones 'Staying Alive' ad for resuscitation or the FAST campaign for spotting a stroke (Face droop, Arm weakness or numbness,
Speech difficulties, Time to phone 999). And sometimes just watching something on television can be a life-saver. I once covered a story
on BBC Radio Bristol about a mum, Marie Lord, at a bus stop spotting the rash of bacterial meningitis in a sick-looking toddler (Able
who'd she'd never met) after seeing Dr Hilary Jones demonstrate the tumbler test on GMTV (the rash doesn't fade when you put
pressure on it). What's great about this story is that she had the kindness to enquire about a stranger's toddler, she used her knowledge to
spot the rash and she had the confidence and courage to act on her
concerns.

'I PULLED UP HIS T-SHIRT AND FROZE, I KNEW IT WAS MENINGITIS'

Marie's Story

'I was waiting for the bus when a woman came over with a baby
slumped over her shoulder. I'll talk to anybody – you do when you're
bored at a bus stop – so I asked if the toddler was tired. She said no,
she thought he had flu. I had a look and his lips and face were a
deathly colour, blue and grey. He was also very floppy. I asked her
whether he had a rash and she said she thought not. I pulled up
Able's T-shirt and there was one on his stomach. I just froze, I knew it
was meningitis. In the ten minutes he was there, the boy had gone
from barely opening his eyes to almost unconscious. There was no

way she had time to wait for the bus and go to the doctor's. I raced
to a phone box. In it was a man I knew. I yanked him out and phoned
for an ambulance.'

Able was unconscious by the time the ambulance arrived, but
received emergency treatment at Bristol Children's Hospital just in
time to save him. His mum Alex said, 'I thought it was just flu. But
when Marie saw the rash, she just dropped her bags and ran to the
phone. I thought she was being a bit dramatic. On the way to the
hospital, Able's decline was rapid. He had to be oxygenated, it was
like he was dying in front of me. If it had been a couple of minutes
later he might not have survived. She saved his life.'

Marie has her own kids but had never seen meningitis before.
'Chicken pox and German measles are the worst I've had to deal
with.'

You can save a life from something you've seen on the television and you
should all know how to spot the signs of meningitis – the NHS website
and any of the meningitis charities provide good information – but
sometimes with sick kids it's a case of trusting your instincts. Sometimes you don't know what the diagnosis is but you know your child is
very ill and you should seek urgent help.

The huge advantage of learning basic life support skills is not just
that you may one day save a life, but you learn how to spot when a
baby, child or adult is in trouble and when to seek help. You get more
confident in acting on your concerns, and being able to explain why
you are concerned and seeking help. You learn to TEA CUP (Think
Explain and Act Correctly Under Pressure), and that knowledge, skills
and confidence will serve you well in other walks of life. You also feel
part of a wider life-saving community where volunteers give back their
time and skills to help others. Giving back to your community is very
good for your mental health and gives your life a deeper sense of meaning and purpose. And of course, the life you save one day may be your
own, or someone you love.

Learning these skills also puts you at a huge advantage in hospital
where you might spot the deterioration of a loved one before the (always
busy) NHS staff. Learning the basic skills of observation – response,

colour, level of consciousness, breathing rate and pulse – and using the confidence you've learned to speak up can save a life even in hospital. One of the commonest causes of avoidable death in the NHS is failure to spot a patient deteriorating in time (e.g. from an infection or sepsis). The observations, skills and courage of a relative can be crucial.

It's not always easy to spot a life-threatening situation. Choking can be quiet, an exhausted asthmatic on the verge of collapse can give up wheezing, and drowning is very rarely like it appears in the movies. Often you have to trust your instincts, and your instincts get better if you have training and gather experience.

'MY DAUGHTER WAS DROWNING AND SHE DIDN'T MAKE A SOUND'

Tom's Story

We were in the pool on holiday and from right across the other side the lifeguard very quickly climbed down from his chair, dived in and started swimming towards us. I was standing next to my wife and I thought, well we're fine, we can all swim, what's he doing? And he was still heading towards us and I looked at my wife and yelled, 'We're fine.' It was all a little embarrassing. And he swam straight past us to where my daughter was swimming. Or rather drowning. She didn't make a sound until he picked her out of the water and then she burst into tears and started screaming, 'Daddy!'

You think when someone is drowning they will wave and splash about and shout for help, but they usually don't. Accidental drowning causes more than 400 deaths in the UK every year, and is the third highest cause of death in children. Many do so within twenty-five yards of a parent or another adult, but it's not always easy to spot. When you're in respiratory distress, your need to breathe often overrides your need to speak. And if your head is slipping in and out of the water, your mouth is rarely above the surface long enough to breathe out, breathe in again and shout for help. You often sink again before you can make yourself heard. You can't wave easily because you put your arms out and press downwards to try to keep yourself above water. Waving makes you go under. And some people can only struggle for less than a minute before they sink.

If you have trained as a lifeguard and you've seen lots of people in distress in the water, you're likely to spot it far more quickly than a parent, even if he or she is a few yards away. Just remember, people who are drowning don't look like they're drowning to people who've only seen it on the TV. Use your eyes and be ever curious. Anyone who can't answer, 'Are you all right?' could be in trouble.

The other great 'aha' moments from learning about what to do in accident and emergency situations are:

You learn that most accidents are preventable. You can then learn to risk-assess your home and use window locks, smoke alarms, carbon monoxide monitors, stair gates, locked medicine cabinets, etc. You can learn to use ladders safely, drive more safely, supervise children even near shallow water, not to let toddlers play with toys they might choke on, and not to leave your sensible head at home when you go on holiday, etc.

You learn there is no such thing as zero risk, and life would be very dull if there was. The skill is to learn to take sensible risks. Don't cross the stupid line. Pause for thought if you aren't sure of a risk. Have the confidence to say no to dropping a tablet of who knows what in a nightclub, or getting in a car with a driver you think might be drunk. Your best chance of being free from illness or accident in future is to moderate your risks and freedoms in the present. Never jump off a bridge without checking the depth of the water. It works in real life and as a metaphor.

Spotting serious illness is about pattern recognition, experience and good luck – looking out for and seeing the red flags – and trusting your instincts. You spend a long time with your loved ones and if you think they're looking really ill, they probably are.

In adults, learn about the signs of heart attack and stroke – prompt action saves lives. Life-threatening illness often comes on quickly or suddenly.

STROKE (advice from Patient.co.uk)

Affects 120,000 people a year. The symptoms of a stroke will depend on the area of the brain that's affected but include sudden . . .

- Weakness of an arm, leg, or both. This may range from total paralysis of one side of the body, to mild clumsiness of one hand.

- Weakness and twisting of one side of the face. This may cause you to drool saliva.

- Problems with balance, coordination, vision, speech, communication, or swallowing.

- Dizziness or unsteadiness.

- Numbness in a part of the body.

- Headache.

- Confusion.

- Loss of consciousness (in severe cases).

Call 999 – prompt treatment may reverse the stroke

HEART ATTACK (Advice from St John Ambulance)

A heart attack is most commonly caused by a sudden blockage of the blood supply to the heart muscle itself – for example, a blood clot. The main risk is that the heart will stop beating.

Look for the sudden onset of . . .

- Persistent central chest pain – often described as vice-like or a heavy crushing pressure.

- Pain spreading (radiating) to the jaw, neck and down one or both arms.

- Breathlessness.

- Discomfort high in the abdomen, similar to indigestion.

- Possible collapse without warning.

- Ashen skin and blueness at the lips.

- Rapid, weak pulse which may be irregular.

- Profuse sweating, skin cold to the touch.

- Gasping for air (air hunger).

- Nausea and/or vomiting.

FIRST AID

- Sit them down in the 'W' position (sitting up at about 75° to the ground with knees bent.

- Call 999/112 for emergency help and tell ambulance control you suspect a heart attack.

- Give an aspirin: if available and not allergic, give them a 300 mg aspirin tablet to chew slowly. It can halve the size of the heart attack. Always worth carrying one in your wallet or purse.

- If they have any medication for angina, such as tablets or a spray, assist them to take it.

- Constantly monitor and record breathing and pulse rate, until help arrives.

- If they become unconscious, give life support. (If you've had no training, think of Vinnie Jones and give chest compressions until the ambulance arrives at the speed of 'Staying Alive'.)

SEPSIS

This is an extreme reaction of the body to infection – and is often missed at home and in hospital. This is a life-threatening condition that arises when the body's response to an infection injures its own tissues and organs. If not picked up and treated quickly, it can lead to shock, multiple organ failure and death. It claims 37,000 lives every year in the UK. That's more than breast cancer, prostate cancer and HIV/AIDS combined. Sepsis often starts with something that seems like flu, gastroenteritis or a chest infection. It can start with what seems like a trivial injury or infection that then spreads. You should seek urgent medical help, or raise concerns for a person already in hospital, if they develop any of the following:

Slurred speech
Extreme shivering or severe muscle pain
Passing no urine in a day
Severe breathlessness
'**I** feel like I might die'
Skin mottled or discoloured

When you get to hospital with sepsis, you need urgent IV antibiotics, IV fluids, oxygen and blood tests. People die avoidably every year, even when they're already in hospital, because sepsis either isn't picked up, or when it is diagnosed vital doses of IV antibiotics are missed or delayed. This is one area where patents and carers must speak up. You must have important drugs on time in hospital, to prevent and treat infection, and to prevent blood clots (DVTs, which can be fatal if they spread to the lungs). And people also die because they sit at home and don't realize they're so ill.

Remember, also, that not everyone with life-threatening illness wants to be treated. Knowing your loved one's wishes towards the end of life, and whether they would rather be cared for at home in familiar surroundings without high-tech intervention, is important.

If you do want treatment, go for a specialist centre – know in advance where the nearest specialist units are for heart disease, cancer and stroke. It doesn't matter what age you are . . .

Sick Kids

Knowing when your baby or child is seriously ill is a challenge for any parent, and you should always trust your instincts and ask for help if you think something isn't right. You don't have to make a diagnosis, just observe your child. Does he or she seem very ill to you? If a baby or child can feed, smile, interact with you and play, it is coping well with its illness. If you have the right information you can make better decisions about when to seek help. The information below is all instantly available on the NHS, NICE and Patient.co.uk websites (with pictures, film clips and more). I am just including it as an example of how the internet can give you the right information when you most need it.

Almost all children with a fever recover quickly and without problems. In a very small proportion of children the fever may not improve or the child's health may worsen, which can sometimes be a sign of a serious illness or infection, such as pneumonia, a urine infection or meningitis.

Fever in babies under three months is rare and can be a sign of serious illness or infection. If your baby is younger than three months and has a fever (38°C or above), or is between three and six months of age with a temperature of 39°C or above, you should seek advice from a healthcare professional.

How to Take the Temperature of a Child

- Don't put a thermometer in the mouth (or bottom) of a child under five.

- Forehead chemical thermometers are unreliable.

- In infants under the age of four weeks, measure body temperature with an electronic thermometer in the armpit.

- In children aged four weeks to five years, measure body temperature by one of the following methods:

  - electronic thermometer in the armpit

  - chemical dot thermometer in the armpit

  - infra-red tympanic thermometer (goes in the ear).

- If you don't have a thermometer, still take note if your child feels hot and feverish.

RED LIGHT SYMPTOMS in your child that you must get urgent help with are:

- Pale/mottled/ashen/blue skin, lips or tongue.

- No response to your voice and play.

- Just looking really ill to you.

- Does not wake, or if roused does not stay awake.

- Weak, high-pitched or continuous cry.

- Grunting.

- Breathing rate greater than sixty breaths per minute in a child aged up to five months; greater than fifty breaths per minute, aged six to twelve months; greater than forty breaths per minute if older than twelve months. Undress your child and time how quickly the chest moves in and out for a minute.

- Sucking in of the muscles in between the ribs as your child breathes (in-drawing), showing they are working really hard to breathe.

- Reduced skin turgor – when you're well, your skin returns quickly to its normal shape if you (gently) squeeze it. If it doesn't, that's a sign of dehydration.

- Bulging fontanelle – feel your baby's soft spot between the skull bones when he or she is well. If it bulges out during illness, that's a red flag sign.

- Children younger than three months with a temperature of 38°C or higher are in a high-risk group for serious illness.

- Children aged three to six months with a temperature of 39°C or higher are in at least 'amber light', and 'red light' if you think they are also unwell.

- Children with a fever lasting more than five days should be assessed for Kawasaki disease.

- Children with a high heart rate are at least an intermediate-risk group for serious illness.

- Cold arms and limbs.

- A weak pulse.

AMBER LIGHT SYMPTOMS you should contact your surgery about are:

- Skin, lips or tongue more pale.

- Not wanting to play.

- Not smiling.

- Wakes only if you make a big, repeated effort to wake him or her.

- Moving less.

- Edges of the nose flare in and out when breathing, showing breathing is harder or faster than normal (nasal flaring).

- Dry mouth and tongue – a sign of dehydration.

- Poor feeding in infants.

- Weeing less/dryer nappies.

- Spikes of very high temperatures (over 39°C), sometimes accompanied by the shakes and sweats.

- A finger or toe 'refill' time of more than three seconds. Squeeze the blood out and see how long it takes to return.

GREEN LIGHT SYMPTOMS that indicate your child will probably get better without medical care:

- Normal colour of skin, lips and tongue.

- Responds normally to your voice and play.

- Content and/or smiling.

- Stays awake or awakens quickly.

- Strong normal cry or not crying.

- Normal skin and eyes.

- Moist mouth and tongue.

Children with fever and any of the symptoms or signs in the red column should be recognized as being at high risk – get help now. Similarly, children with fever and any of the amber symptoms or signs and none in the red column are at intermediate risk – tell your GP. Children with fever and the signs in the green column and none in the amber or red columns are at low risk and you can start by caring for them yourself and calling for help if amber or red symptoms appear. Always tell your doctor if you have travelled abroad recently, and where.

A colour traffic light table is available from the NICE website. There are apps to help spot sick kids too. The bottom line is that you know your child best, and are the best judge to say if he or she is ill. Trust your instincts and have the confidence to seek an opinion sooner rather than later, and urgently for red flag signs.

NOTE: You should also monitor your children with the traffic light system when they're in hospital. Don't assume the busy staff will always spot a deterioration. If you spot a red flag symptom or sign in hospital, point it out urgently. The same applies to adults. To repeat, one of the most common reasons patients come to avoidable harm in hospitals is that a treatable deterioration in their condition is either not spotted or not acted on swiftly.

THE RIGHT WAY TO USE GP SERVICES

Booking an Urgent Appointment

Serious illnesses often (but not always) come on fairly quickly or even suddenly, and may involve a change or 'red flag' that points to the need for an urgent appointment. In an emergency, don't waste time phoning your GP. Dial 999. Red flags don't always mean serious illness – in fact, usually they don't – but they increase your odds of a serious illness enough to warrant seeing a GP as soon as you can (e.g. abnormal bleeding from anywhere, a persistent change in pooing or peeing habits, loss of appetite, weight, movement, coordination, sensation, vision, speech or hearing, difficulty swallowing, turning yellow, blackouts, falls, night sweats, lumps and bumps, pain and headaches especially if it wakes you at night or you wake with it in the morning). Macmillan (www.macmillan.org.uk) do a very clear 'symptoms and signs of cancer' guide you should read and act on (it tells you when to see your GP urgently). The NICE website gives clear guidance on what symptoms and signs need a cancer referral, usually with a two-week wait. You can find excllent advice at www.patient.co.uk and www.nhs.uk (try the Map of Medicine guidelines).

If you do have cancer, your chances of survival and returning to a good quality of life depend on a long chain of events starting with you spotting your symptoms and asking for help, to your GP investigating and referring you to the right specialist, to the hospital being able to see, investigate, diagnose and treat you swiftly and correctly. Delays or errors at any stage can affect your chances, but they will inevitably happen sometimes in an organization as under pressure as the NHS. Often, it may be left to you to spot errors, get other opinions, chase results and appointments and voice your concerns. Once you've got over the shock of a serious diagnosis, try to find the energy to wise up and get as involved as you can.

Booking Non-Urgent Appointments

If your appointment isn't urgent, you have time to seek advice from the NHS and Patient.co.uk websites, from friends and family and from your local pharmacist, who may offer a surprising number of services but also direct you to your GP if he or she thinks you need a medical or nursing opinion. The vast majority of non-urgent symptoms get better in time, and many can be safely assessed over the phone.

Access and Organize Your Own Medical Records

Your records may be full of vital information, littered with errors or much duller than you'd hoped. But the principle of understanding, organizing and controlling your data and records in a way that is useful to you is important, particularly if you have to use the NHS a lot. The more complex your care, the higher the potential risks, rewards and chances of error. Keeping copies of all the important letters written about you across the NHS and social care, in date order, gives you a fascinating picture of what the system thinks is wrong with you and what it thinks you need. It may be very different from your own view, or absolutely spot on. Either way, it's worth knowing and sharing the file with others as you move around this vast organization.

Learn About How the Practice Works, What Services It Offers, and How It Fits in with the Local NHS

The practice website is a good place to start. If you're choosing a new practice or GP, you can visit, see if you can easily walk or park, chat through what it offers with the practice manager, and ask friends and family what their experiences are. Online ratings by patients are theoretically useful, but as yet haven't been used in large enough numbers to be reliable. It's always worth feeding back your experiences and suggestions for better care to your practice, or via your patient participation group (PPG).

Can You Sort Your Problem out Over the Phone, Email, Skype or Online?

I had a brilliant physiotherapy service over the phone. I told the physio all about my shoulder pain, she asked me questions, got me to move my arm as much as I could in various directions and then recommended a series of exercises. We did a follow up on the phone to and my shoulder is now completely better without needing to see anyone. It made me wonder how many other symptoms could be sorted out over the phone.

Bev, forty-nine

Often you need advice but not necessarily a consultation, and most GP practices offer phone consultations, or a call-back service that sorts out half the problems there and then (hint: make sure the practice has an up-to-date number to call you back on). Some GPs use Skype and other smartphone apps, and some are now consulting by email and using text services to monitor diseases and motivate you to manage them better.

In Airedale, West Yorkshire, care home residents have tele-access to doctors from the local NHS hospital over a secure video link. They love it, they get the advice they need and their hospital admissions have almost halved. Many problems can be sorted out without face-to-face consultations, but you have to accept the slight risk that no system is completely secure. However, email consulting is a lot more safe and secure that those tatty old envelopes we used to try to cram all your vital records into and then mix them all up with other patients' records. And emails and texts are a lot easier to read than a doctor's handwriting. GP practices vary enormously in their desire to embrace new technology, so you may have to ask around to find one that does. I email my blood pressure readings and get blood results and advice back by email.

For non-urgent problems, the NHS, Patient.co.uk, healthtalk.org, Embarrassing Bodies and Embarrassing Problems websites may have the answers you need. If you already have a diagnosis, a good charity provides the combination of accurate information, support and advice.

Is the Practice Nurse a Better Bet Than a GP?

Practice nurses are now in charge of most of the long-term diseases (e.g. heart disease, asthma, diabetes, depression), they do immunizations, wound dressings, health checks, contraception and stop-smoking advice. They can also offer you help to monitor illnesses on your own at home using devices that send data via your computer or mobile phone (e.g. the Flo system), saving you countless trips to the surgery, giving you control and independence and even reducing hospital admissions. You can get text reminders to measure your blood sugar, take your tablets and get updates on blood results and investigations without going to the surgery. A good nurse, like a good GP, can be the gold dust you need to get the right NHS care. And great company too.

Know What Care You Should Be Getting

For just about every mental and physical illness, and for social care, there are agreed standards of care that you should be getting, and clear information written for patients and carers on the NICE website – www.nice.org.uk; www.htmc.co.uk is also worth a look. Spend time getting to know the standard of care you should be getting – e.g. if you have any chronic disease, you should have a care plan you have agreed to and understood, with clear instructions as to what to do if your illness flares up. Many patients don't have this and don't even know they're entitled to it. Once you know what care you should be getting, you can figure out how much you can do for yourself and what you need help with. And asking for help is a lot easier when you know what you're talking about.

Know What Care and Choices You Might Expect

The healthtalk.org website is simply superb. You can find information on a range of illnesses and other health-related issues through seeing and hearing people's real-life experiences. Thousands of people have shared their experiences on film to help others understand what it's really like to have a health condition such as breast cancer or arthritis. There are films to watch, transcripts to read – all real, all from patients like you. It's an essential website for NHS staff and patients. If you want to read about the standards of care you should be getting for any particular illness, try the Quality Standards on the NICE website.

Out of Hours

Politicians are fond of promising a seven-day NHS, where the lights are always on and your chances of survival are the same whatever day, or time of the day or night, you happen to get sick. It isn't going to happen soon. You shouldn't be blamed for going to an emergency department if you can't get care elsewhere – there shouldn't be a 'wrong door' policy in the NHS. Your local NHS should have a Choose Well website to guide you to the choices available to you, and what you can do to self-care. For an example, check out the excellent website www. choosewellmanchester.org.uk. Good information often buys you time. In general . . .

- For red flag/emergency signs and symptoms in children and adults dial 999.

- If you're not sure, dial 111 out of hours but try your GP first during the day. You may well be directed to 111, or a GP may guarantee to phone you back within twenty minutes and visit you within an hour.

- If you know you have a walk-in or urgent care centre locally, walk in. Walk-in centres are not for heart attacks, strokes or other emergencies.

- A good chemist can treat a surprising number of ailments and offer good advice. Always worth trying.

- Sexual health clinics don't require an appointment – although they encourage you to make one if you can. If you need emergency contraception, the sooner you take it after sex the better. It's worth trying up to 120 hours after sex. You can buy if from a chemist if you can't quickly get it free from the NHS.

- If you can't get through to your GP or convince the receptionist an emergency assessment is needed, and the patient is worsening, phone 999 or go directly to an emergency department.

- If your symptoms are serious or won't go, SCAN them (see below).

The NHS and Patient.co.uk websites have useful symptom sorters to help you think about what the diagnosis might be, whether you need to seek help or whether you can wait and see if they go. If symptoms are persisting, it's worth doing a SCAN on them to figure out if you need a GP appointment and why. Talk it through with a friend, member of your family or pharmacist.

> **S**ymptoms, **S**tory and **S**elf-care
> **C**oncerns
> **A**ssessment
> **N**eeds

SYMPTOMS, STORY and **SELF-CARE** . . . What are your symptoms and what is your story? Write down your symptoms in the order they occurred, think about their severity, how they may have changed and if anything makes them better or worse. What self-care have you tried already? Your past medical history, medications, lifestyle and circumstances can also be crucial to getting the right diagnosis. Symptom diaries are very useful to track how symptoms vary over time. Is anything happening in your life or work that might be causing or contributing to your symptoms?

CONCERNS . . . What are your concerns? Until these are addressed and acknowledged, you will keep worrying. You should try to say what your main concern is early in any consultation. Writing it down can help.

ASSESSMENT . . . What is your assessment of the problem? What do you think the cause, or causes may be? Use the websites above to help you sort through your symptoms if you want to. They will guide you as to how quickly you need to seek NHS help, or whether you can wait and see if symptoms settle. Friends, families, charities and chat rooms can also be useful sources of support to help you accurately assess and deal with a problem. You don't have to make the diagnosis, and you won't always be right if you do. Many doctors get a little prickly if you appear to be doing our job, but in my experience, a patient's assessment of their situation is more often right than wrong. If your thoughts don't match your doctor's, ask, 'What else might it be?' or 'Have you considered this diagnosis?'

NEEDS . . . What are your needs? The NHS is founded on treatment according to need, and yet very rarely in the NHS do doctors remember to ask you what your needs are, or do patients tell us, whereas in the social care system, you talk about needs all the time. If you're worried that saying, 'This is what I need' sounds needy, you could say, 'This is what I want' or – less pushy – 'This is what I hoped for from this consultation' or 'this is what matters most to me.' Either way, get your needs, wants or hopes on that ten-minute table. Many patients want the reassurance of an expert opinion more than a prescription, and if that's the case let your GP know. Otherwise you might get a prescription without much of an explanation. Everyone needs the most accurate diagnosis possible in the circumstances, a choice of treatments that are proven to be effective and a safety net if symptoms persist or worsen. And always ask, 'What is likely to happen if we did nothing?'

NOTE: I once worked in a practice where the patients' symptoms and concerns were noted when they made the appointment (with their consent), and the doctor could see these in advance. It made a huge difference to the smooth running of the consultations because the doctor's brain started clicking into gear earlier and the agenda for the consultation was agreed in advance. Patients were also allowed to choose between five-, ten- and twenty-minute appointments, and they generally chose very wisely.

GP consultations barely last ten minutes, although you can try to book a double appointment for complex problems. Many specialist appointments are only fifteen minutes in the NHS (longer privately). It's a ridiculously short time to practise safe, high-quality medicine, so it's worth giving some thought to getting the most out of your perilously short time.

Getting the Most From a Consultation

Luke's Story

My sister swears that a mixture of humour and self-deprecation is the best way to lightly challenge doctors and check they are not about to make a terrible mistake with her children. She says something like: 'Can I ask you some questions so I'm not worrying at 3am and Googling it instead of talking to a proper doctor? Consider it a service to my mental health as well to the health of my children.'

Nigel's Story

When I go to see any doctor, I get very nervous. So I imagine I'm George Clooney. Confident, cool, assertive but never irritating. I don't tell anyone what I'm doing – that would be ridiculous. But I've found people take more notice of me and seem to listen when I'm imagining I'm George. I'm not pretending to be him, just drawing on his confidence.

Arrive in good time, but bring a good book and a copy of your SCAN, or at least a note of your main concern and what you most want or need from the consultation.

The NHS is built on human relationships and they're a two-way street. Getting to know the names of the staff in your practice, looking them in the eye, smiling and asking how they are can go a long way to prompting them to do the same to you, even though they may be buckling under the workload. Working as a team with the frontline staff is your best chance of making sense of, and surviving, the NHS.

Handshake and Hello

Consider starting every consultation by shaking the hand firmly of whoever you're consulting with, look them in the eye and say, 'Hello'. This is important for a number of reasons:

- It makes you connect with each other at the start of the consultation. Touch, eye contact, body language, speech and tone of voice are all very revealing.

- Often doctors are typing up the previous patient's notes as you enter. Putting your hand out and leaving it there until it's shaken is a good way of getting them to focus away from the computer back on to you.

- Some NHS staff will always shake your hand, smile, look you in the eye and say, 'Hello, my name is . . .' if you haven't met them before, but not all. The wonderful Dr Kate Granger made great strides in encouraging every NHS worker to do this (see later), but patients can also take the initiative and start with a handshake, eye contact and introduction. It makes the consultation a meeting between experts from the outset. You're an expert in your illness and how you live your life, your doctor is an expert in trying to improve your life.

- If you're anxious about seeing a doctor, as most of us are, you can relieve some of that anxiety by adopting confident behaviours. A firm handshake may even improve your self-confidence by setting the tone at the start of the consultation.

Some doctors and patients are fearful of shaking hands because of the risk of passing on infections, but you can (and should) wash them afterwards. I once met a patient who washed his hands in my sink and then asked me to do the same, before he shook my hand. If your culture does not permit handshaking, think of other ways of connecting with your doctor. An early question is often worth trying, and hard to ignore. 'How are you today, doctor?'

What Happens in a Consultation?

Just as you can take your own SCAN into a consultation, your GP and nurse will do an extended version for themselves when they see you.

In just ten minutes, a GP has to run SCANS:

> **S**ymptoms and **S**tory
> **C**onnect
> **A**ssess, **A**cknowledge and **A**gree
> **N**egotiate and assess **N**eeds
> **S**ummarize and agree a **S**afety net

SYMPTOMS and **STORY** . . . Listen to your symptoms and story.

CONNECT . . . With you as a person.

ASSESS . . . Your symptoms, story and needs, **ACKNOWLEDGE** your concerns and feelings, and **AGREE** the nature of the problems with you – what can be sorted out today and what may have to wait.

NEGOTIATE . . . A plan to improve your life/investigate further based on the most likely diagnosis and your **NEEDS**.

SUMMARIZE . . . The plan, check you've both understood it and ask if you have any questions. Finally, agree a **SAFETY NET** with you if symptoms persist or worsen.

That's a hell of a lot to do in ten minutes, and it may be better to focus on one symptom or problem (or set of symptoms and related problems) in detail, than do a scatter gun approach for multiple problems.

A few doctors will put a note up saying '1 problem only' and I even met one who had an egg timer that went off when your ten minutes was up. There is never enough time in the NHS. If you have a serious problem that needs time, book a double appointment. Illnesses evolve over time and no-one gets everything right first time so you may need several consultations, or your own research, to sort out a persistent problem.

I used the SCANS template to help teach medical students how to communicate with patients as a lecturer at Birmingham and Bristol universities. The first-year students were often very kind and great listeners, but lacked confidence because they lacked knowledge. Older students had more knowledge but were sometimes more controlling and worse listeners. After a few years, I realized that patients need coaching to talk to doctors as much as the other way round, which is partly what this book is about. Confident patients often get better care, but confidence comes with education, training, knowledge and success. You also need to accept fear and learn from failure. The self-knowledge of your own SCAN is a good start. If you want to go on to www.nice.org.uk and find out what care you're entitled to and to what standard for just about every illness, it will build your knowledge and confidence further. Many charity websites are also a goldmine of support and information.

Good GPs go through their SCANS stages seamlessly and seemingly effortlessly, although their brains are working overtime to make sure they haven't missed anything that could prove to be important or even fatal; another part of their brain is outside hovering over the fifteen patients they still have to see. The pressure is often on to make a diagnosis or come up with a management plan in a short space of time. Getting your SCAN to the doctor in advance could make all the difference between a great and an unsatisfactory consultation. If your doctor does provide email access, you might be able to send your SCAN when booking your appointment. Your previous SCANs could be grouped together as a symptom diary. This may be an easier way to get to grips with your care than reading your electronic records, which aren't often organized in a way that patients can quickly understand. If you are an app developer, feel free to experiment with the SCAN idea.

In the meantime, it's worth taking a couple of copies of your SCAN in with you, one for you to add notes to, and one to leave with the GP or nurse to refer to. It shouldn't be a long, rambling list but a thoughtful attempt by you to nail your concerns and needs in advance and get the most out of your ten minutes. Put your main concern at the top!

Other Consultation Tips – these tips come from an audience in Harrogate

I've got a really complicated disease that I don't fully understand – I was told I had epilepsy originally, which was a shock, but now they think there's something wrong with my heart that was making me faint and it could actually stop all together, which is an even bigger shock. I don't really like to dwell on it, I'm on some drugs and I get panicky when I have to go to hospital which makes me worry that my pulse will go up and my heart is going to stop. And I never remember anything the doctors say, or at least I've forgotten by the time I get home. I take my wife but we always disagree on what was said. Then I got the idea of recording every consultation on my phone. Some doctors don't like it, most are fine when I say it's for me and my family, not the *Daily Mail*. And I think their explanations are better when they know they're being recorded. I take it away with me and we listen back again away from the stress of the hospital. I make a few notes and now my treatment is a lot better and I think I know what I'm doing. And so does my wife.

I always dress up to see the doctor – I'm sure you're taken more seriously if you look more important. When my mother was ill and we couldn't get any answers, I actually glammed up to see the consultant. Pitiful, I know, but I'm sure it worked.

I always carry a good book with me when I use the NHS. Something intellectual. It subtly lets everyone know that I'm intelligent and I want to be treated that way and included in my care.

I always check the ear pieces when I see a GP. If they've got someone else's wax in them, then they're not coming near me.

I have a multi-purpose NHS T-shirt that says 'Please include me in all decisions about my care.' It lets everyone know what kind of patient I am immediately. If I'm knackered and I just want to be looked after, I don't wear it.

It's up to you whether you want to prepare for a consultation in advance or just turn up and wing it. You can dress up, carry the book, wear the T-shirt, bring the list or just turn up. You should hopefully agree on an action plan during the consultation. If you don't, and you're worried, seek a second opinion. Those who seek other opinions are sometimes amazed at how different they can be. Getting the same second opinion can be both frustrating and reassuring.

If you do get a second opinion, it should be judged on your concerns and not biased by what a previous doctor has said. Doctors have an unfortunate habit of just doing or saying what the previous doctor did or said. Getting a second opinion is tough enough; you need to make sure it's looked at with fresh eyes. Some illnesses are hard to diagnose in the early stages, and the initial diagnosis is sometimes wrong. Always ask, 'What else could it be?' 'How would I know?' and 'What should I do if it doesn't get better?'

Try not to waste your ten minutes talking about stuff that doesn't really matter to you, then say what really does matter right at the very end with your hand on the door handle. Your GP is not a mind reader but should be a kind listener. You sometimes have to be brave to talk about a difficult subject such as depression or abuse, especially with a new doctor. Showing a concern written down in advance can be a good way in. It may be easier to write it down than say it.

Do expect to be examined, so dress accordingly. Loose clothes are best and not too many layers. If they're smart too, your GP might take you more seriously (we should treat you by need, not appearance, but the NHS sometimes gives better care to those who dress up to see the doctor).

If you're a woman and might need an internal examination, go between periods, not in the middle of one.

If you've got kids, see if you could leave them with someone, so the ten minutes is all about you and not disrupted.

If you think you have a urine infection, take a mid-stream sample in a clean jar. It will save time.

Show your GP anything apart from your pets or your teeth.

As well as taking notes into a consultation, you can make notes while you're there. Many mobile phones have a record facility and your GP shouldn't mind if you record your consultation for your personal use and to educate your carers too. You can take a friend in too. Most people forget most of what was said in a consultation so it makes perfect sense to *write it down or record it* (WIDORI).

If you've thought about your needs in advance, and your GP agrees, you can then move on to how likely any treatment is to help you meet them. If you share in decisions about your care, you're likely to get better care that's right for you. To make a good choice, you must let your doctor know your hopes and fears, what matters most to you in your life and what you must avoid. You also need to know the risks, benefits and likely success rates of the possible treatments. And it's always worth asking, 'What if we did nothing?' The body has evolved an extraordinary capacity to heal itself in time.

At the end of every consultation, check:

- What is my main problem?

- What do I need to do now?

- Why is it important for me to do this?

- What if it doesn't get better?

Take a few moments after the consultation to write the answers down or update your SCAN with the agreed plan of action and safety net. Otherwise you'll forget what was said surprisingly quickly. If you recorded your consultation on your phone, you can listen back to it when you get home over a cup of tea.

A lot of decisions don't need to be made there and then, and if you're committing yourself to surgery or drugs for life, it's worth taking time over that decision and not rushing it in a consultation. See also the section on The Right Decision for You.

The kind of questions you need to ask yourself are:

- What are my options?

- What are the pros and cons of each option for me?

- How do I get support to help me make a decision that is right for me?

- What is likely to happen if we did nothing?

- What if we can't agree on a referral?

If you think you need a specialist referral but your GP doesn't, ask and write down the reasons why. It may be that you disagree on the diagnosis, in which case ask for his or her reasoning and evidence that led to the diagnosis, and what else it might be. Ask what the safety plan is that might trigger a referral. The more research you do, the more likely you are to have a more equal conversation. The NICE website, for example, gives clear guidance on what symptoms and signs need a cancer referral, usually with a two-week wait. The Macmillan website also gives clear advice on spotting cancer early. Writing down your doctor's reasoning is not about proving him or her wrong, but knowing how that decision was reached. If you still don't understand or disagree, get a second opinion, particularly if it's clear to you that you meet the criteria for an urgent referral. It doesn't matter where your child's meningitis is suspected (at the surgery, in casualty, in the queue for the bus stop). What matters is that once it has been suspected, it is investigated urgently. Some doctors still don't believe in certain diagnoses, for example chronic fatigue syndrome/ME, even though it clearly exists and NICE has issued clear guidance on diagnosis and specialist referral. In instances like this, and indeed all instances when you're struggling to be taken seriously or to get a referral, the advice from a charity can be gold dust (see later).

Your risk of serious illness depends on your genes, habits, age and illnesses you've had already. Just because you've had one cancer, you might think it would be very bad luck to have another, but it is possible. Some cancers increase your risk of getting others, and because cancer treatment has improved so much, people are living longer with their first cancer and so their chances of getting another ironically go up. Again, a specialist charity website like Macmillan will help you understand what you are most at risk of and what you can do about it.

Medicine is an imperfect science, and people (including NHS staff) live complex and messy lives that give them all sorts of symptoms, some of which are – and remain – medically unexplained. There's sometimes a payoff between having lots of investigations and referrals, and accepting that there are some symptoms that we currently can't diagnose or fully explain. Learning to live well within the limits of these symptoms can be tough, but it's often better than being aboard a rollercoaster of medical investigations with no clear goals and no obvious end in sight. Medical interventions are often a lot less powerful and effective than you'd think, and it's surprisingly easy to do more harm than good. Which is why you should always ask, 'What is likely to happen if we did nothing?' The likely, but not guaranteed, answer is that you'll live to eighty. Friendship, community, curiosity, activity and being absorbed by what interests you is often far more life-enhancing than anything your GP can offer.

Be a Chaser

If you've had tests, X-rays, scans or a hospital referral, chase them up. Think of it as your responsibility to keep your care on track. Like all complex health services, the NHS is littered with errors, and even more are waiting to happen. Blood results and pathology reports sometimes get misfiled, and sometimes a chance to make a diagnosis or pick up a disease before it causes more harm is lost. Referrals can also get lost somewhere between GP-land and hospital, or between hospital departments. Chase them up. Let them know you're still alive and waiting. Give them your phone number for a last-minute cancellation slot. Chase, chase, chase.

Of course, if you had electronic access to all your medical records, test results and important letters from home, you wouldn't have to do so much chasing. Electronic access to part of your NHS GP records has been promised this year (2015). We shall see. Might be worth chasing.

Don't Die of Embarrassment

Before the NHS can treat a serious illness, you – or your friends or family – have to recognize when you're seriously ill. Sometimes, you can push and punish your mind and body so much you don't realize you've got red flag symptoms, or you may just choose to deny them. Admitting you're ill can be as hard as admitting you have an addiction, and you may have to overcome fear, stigma and embarrassment. Or you may just be so busy you don't have time to be ill.

Some people die of embarrassment rather than seek help for treatable cancers. Many more have done themselves serious harm by not seeking help quickly. Cancer can pop up in the most embarrassing places but the sooner you seek help for blood loss, lumps, sores, severe pain, yellow skin or weight loss, the better. Anything that wakes you at night (e.g. pain or sweats) needs checking out, as does any unpleasant symptom you wake up with in the morning (e.g. headaches or nausea). Sudden loss of anything is a medical emergency (e.g. sight, feeling, movement, consciousness), as is sudden onset of chest pain, breathing difficulties or the worst headache ever. You don't have to make a diagnosis, but you do have to dial 999 and if you're trained in life support, you can save a life.

Many cancers are now curable but only if you come forward to be cured. I once met a man who let his testicle swell to 15cm – larger than a grapefruit – because he was embarrassed at having a lump down there and, as it got bigger, he was worried that his GP would think he was an idiot for sitting on it for so long. It wasn't until it really pressed on the nerve endings that he sought help. He survived his cancer but lost a testicle that might well have been saved if he'd come earlier.

Another man asked for a visit when the pain in his testicles was so severe, he fainted. The pain had been excruciating for four hours, and he had a torsion on both sides – a twisting of the tissue that fixes the testicles in the scrotum. It can lead to irreversible damage if it isn't swiftly untwisted under anaesthetic.

His delay in asking for help also cost him a testicle.

The cycle of delay caused by embarrassment, not knowing, fear, stoicism and misplaced optimism is common throughout medicine. It causes huge suffering and occasionally death, and isn't always easy to predict. Some people are ashamed at having a sexually transmitted infection, and many don't realize they have because they have no symptoms. Some people are afraid of revealing a breast lump or rectal bleeding. Embarrassment and fear can be barriers in just about every chronic disease (epilepsy, asthma, diabetes), particularly if you're overweight. As one of my doctor friends confided, 'I've just let a shoe assistant sell me completely the wrong shade of polish. The mistake was obvious but I didn't say anything because she'll just think, "Silly fat cow, what does she know?"' If overweight doctors are too shy to buy the right shoe shine, imagine how hard people find it to access the NHS?

There are two great websites – Embarrassing Bodies and Embarrassing Problems – that will help you tackle and seek help for just about any problem, no matter how embarrassing it seems to you now. Remember too that many doctors and nurses have pretty much seen it all – we're not shocked by much, and we're good at dealing with awkward issues. Choose the person in your practice you find it easiest to talk to.

What If I Don't Get on with My GP?

Healthcare works best when patients, carers and staff all feel part of the same team, working towards the same goals. If you don't get on with your GP, see another if you can. You are entitled to, and it will benefit you both in the long term. If you find a GP you get on with, stick with him or her. A great GP is one of the best chances you have of getting great NHS care. He or she will protect you from unnecessary tests and referrals, but refer you to hospital when you really need it. Work as a partner with your GP, take control of as much of your health as you can, give honest feedback, check you're getting the right care and speak up if you have any concerns. And if you can make each other laugh, that's a huge bonus.

THE RIGHT DIAGNOSIS

Ralph's Story

I felt bloody awful for months, tired, depressed, falling asleep in front
of the TV as soon as I got home. Great big bags under my eyes. I
looked it up on the internet and thought it was my thyroid. I didn't
tell my GP I'd looked it up but she said, 'I think it might be your
thyroid.' So I had the blood test. And it was completely normal.
Turned out I had sleep apnoea and now I've had some specialist
treatment, sleep with prongs up my nose and lost a bit of weight, I
feel great. I still look things up on the internet, I just realize it won't
always be right. And neither will my GP. But we got there in the end.
I just knew how I felt wasn't normal and I needed help.

Heather's Story

My son had a lump on his back – it didn't hurt when you pressed it
but it was quite firm and it didn't go away and kept slowly growing.
The GP thought it was probably just fat, but there was a small chance
it could be something more serious so we should watch and wait. I
didn't want to watch and wait. I looked up the NICE guidelines for
suspected cancer. We ticked three of the boxes, and you only had
to tick two. So I asked for a referral and got it. It was cancer. We were
seen in two weeks on the NHS and we got it before it spread. The
treatment was great but to get an early referral I felt I needed to find
out what the criteria were, what we were entitled to and to ask for it.

Mike's Story

I felt a bit unwell and got this odd patch of red skin on my chest, and
then I got loads of little red blobs all over my body. I looked it up on
the Patient.co.uk website and it sounded like Pityriasis rosea, which I
had no idea how to pronounce, but it looked exactly like it did in the
photo and was described in the information sheet. And I got a
second opinion from the NHS website which said the same – I
probably had a harmless but horrible looking skin thing, that would
get better on its own – but it also said I should see my GP to confirm

the diagnosis. I'd have to take half a day off work to do that, so I emailed him a photo with my symptoms. He agreed and we did nothing, but it took six weeks to go.

Imran's Story

I had chest pain – not awful, but I'd never had it before. I'm fit, don't smoke, no family history – thought it had to be indigestion. It wasn't bad enough to need to go to hospital, but it wasn't going with antacid so I went to see my GP. He was on it like a flash. Blue light, straight into hospital. I didn't want to go – lots of work on – but he insisted. Paramedics did an ECG, said I'd had a heart attack and took me straight to the hospital catheter lab. I could watch my own angiogram. It bloody hurt. I know a bit about the heart so I said, 'Aren't there supposed to be three coronary arteries?' There were only two showing, and one was completely blocked. The cardiologist put a stent in it while I was watching – that takes some balls – and the pain went immediately. He told me afterwards that the blockage I had was known as 'the widow-maker'. It was unblocked within two hours of my GP spotting it. The NHS can be amazing in an emergency.

There are three great advantages to finding out how the body works, and how it goes wrong. You can understand why and how many diseases can be prevented, you might help nail the right diagnosis early on before too much damage is done and you can understand how you or indeed any doctor will never always get the right diagnosis, right first time. A good place to start is a great book by the anatomist and broadcaster Dr (now Professor) Alice Roberts called *Don't Die Young*. Although you need very good A levels to get into medical school, most of medicine isn't rocket science – it isn't that hard to understand how diseases occur. However, spotting them isn't always easy.

Let's take bowel cancer as an example.

Bowel cancer occurs in the colon and the rectum. The colon is a tube that's 150cm long, and goes up the right-hand side of your abdomen, across the top and then down the left-hand side, where it joins the rectum (15cm long), which stores poo before it's passed out from the anus.

Bowel (colo-rectal) cancer can occur anywhere along this tube. It usually starts as a small polyp, like a tiny bump, with no symptoms, which is why screening to pick up and remove polyps can be a life-saver, although many don't become cancerous. Polyps can bleed enough to be picked up on a test of your poo, but not enough to see it when you poo.

As the cancer grows, the symptoms that develop can vary, depending on how far the cancer is along the colon.

If it's on the left-hand side, on the way down to the anus, it's more likely that you will have symptoms and that it will be picked up earlier. This is because any bleeding is likely to be seen in or before your poo and as the polyp grows into the tube you can get a feeling of wanting to pass a poo (your colon mistakes the polyp for poo) but not being able to. It can also block the poo coming out so your pattern of pooing changes – you can either become constipated and not pass much, or only liquid poo can get past it and you have diarrhoea, and sometimes pass mucous – clear fluid from the lining of the bowel that doesn't easily flush away because you're really pushing hard to get the polyp out. You often get pain that comes and goes (colicky) and sometimes a hard lump on the left-hand side of your abdomen.

If the polyp pokes into the tube of your colon on the right-hand side, far away from the anus, it's harder to diagnose. You may only get a little, if any, pain and any bleeding may not show up by the time it comes out of the anus (apart from on a test of your poo). It's less likely to change the frequency or type of your poos, and less likely to block them. You may get weight loss and tiredness (from anaemia caused by the blood loss, and the general effect of cancer) but these symptoms happen with lots of other diseases too. So an early diagnosis is harder.

Finally, there are other diseases that can cause severe bowel symptoms: diverticular disease, inflammatory bowel disease, irritable bowel syndrome, haemorrhoids, infection, blockage of the blood vessels. So no doctor (or patient) is going to get the diagnosis right every time.

The same uncertainties happen in every serious diagnosis. The more hidden away a part of the body is (e.g. ovary, pancreas), the harder it can be to diagnose cancer early. Most diseases are more common as you get older, but don't be falsely reassured just because you are young. Severe symptoms that aren't going away need investigating.

One of the strongest arguments for participating in your care is that the NHS won't always get all your treatment right first time, from start to finish. All human beings make errors every day, and in an NHS under pressure and understaffed, with demand exceeding supply, errors are all too common. Patients and carers may spot them happening, or about to happen, but it takes confidence and courage to speak up. Don't be afraid. Stopping harm in its tracks could save your life or the life of someone you love.

Difficult diagnoses can rarely be done in ten minutes. GPs are under incessant pressure to manage demand and help balance the books. There is huge pressure not to refer to hospital because of financial pressures, making it far too easy to make a serious error. As in many parts of the NHS, there is no safety net. That's why I don't agree with political proposals to publicly 'out' GPs for not investigating diseases sooner by putting a red flag next to their name or practice on the NHS website. This could have a devastating effect on hospital referrals and on the mental health of GPs, and encourage doctors to hide errors rather than admit to them and learn from them.

Most people, at some stage in their life, will get a complex, chronic disease, but no-one will get the right diagnosis first time, every time. There are all sorts of delays in the diagnoses of many of these diseases, but no evidence that blaming GPs on the brink of a breakdown will improve the care that patients get. There is no reason, however, for you not to do some research and suggest, 'Could it be this?' 'If not, why not?' and keep a record of the answers for your own notes.

Around 60 per cent of negligence claims against GPs are related to a failure to diagnose. Some are down to 'system errors', such as the misfiling of a test result, which is why it's so important to chase up the results of any tests you have, and not to assume that no news is good news.

But most errors in diagnosis are down to 'thinking errors'. These include:

- Anchoring bias - locking on to a diagnosis too soon and failing to consider all the evidence or adjust to new information.

- Availability bias - thinking that a similar recent presentation you have encountered is also happening in the present situation. You've had bleeding haemorrhoids before so that's what it is this time, rather than bowel cancer.

- Confirmation bias – we only seek out evidence that supports our pre-conceived opinion and don't look for evidence that would prove it wrong.

- Diagnosis momentum – we accept the previous diagnosis of another doctor without challenging it rigorously.

- Overconfidence bias – we think we know best and over-rely on our own ability, intuition and judgement rather than the evidence.

- Premature closure – we jump to a conclusion because we have to get you out of the room in ten minutes.

- Search-satisfying bias – a 'eureka' moment, possibly down to something we spot on Google, that stops all further thought on the matter.

The most common thinking error among doctors is 'anchoring bias' – where doctors may jump to premature conclusions by assuming that they're thinking about things in the right context when they may not be. They may then fail to undertake a broader search for other possibilities. Common things are common, we place our money on the most likely and move on.

If you have a rare disease, you may well be misdiagnosed several (even many) times. Most doctors will initially opt for the most likely diagnosis and try to close the deal in ten minutes unless he or she is nudged towards something rarer. We often forget to ask if you have travelled abroad, for example, so your fever may well be put down to a cold unless you volunteer that you were recently working in West Africa, which opens up the possibility of a tropical disease and would currently raise the alarm of Ebola.

Making the right diagnosis means having the time to keep testing different hypotheses as bits of the jigsaw fall into place, and it may only unfold over several consultations as more evidence emerges to support a different train of thought. And quite often, people have messy, complicated lives with deeply unpleasant symptoms but no known diagnosis. You may have to live without a diagnosis, and even if you have one it's only any use if it helps you improve or understand your life and how you're feeling.

Diagnosis can be made harder by the fact that patients often see different doctors and don't always tell us the truth. Recently, a sixteen-year-old woman won an out-of-court settlement from a GP after he failed to diagnose she was pregnant. She went on to deliver a healthy baby but developed post-natal depression, and raised a claim against her GP arguing that, had she known she was pregnant, she would have requested a termination.

She went to the GP with symptoms of vomiting and saying her periods had stopped, but denied having had sex and a pregnancy test was not carried out. The patient had also presented on several occasions to out-of-hours services and other GPs complaining of the same symptoms. An existing three-year history of sinusitis was assumed to be the cause of her nausea and vomiting. A period of three months then passed during which several consultations took place, before a home pregnancy test proved to be positive. It seems odd when confronted with a sixteen-year-old on several occasions having missed periods that no-one asked if they might do a pregnancy test, but the patient had denied having sex. Unsurprisingly, however, she denied it because her mother was in the room.

A switched-on doctor might not ask clumsy sex questions in front of your mother, and would find a way of separating you. But another message here is that you have a right to see a doctor or nurse with a relative in support *or* on your own. It's your choice, and if there's something you need to say to help the doctor make the right diagnosis, but not in front of your mother, you need to find a way of passing that information on. It could be a private note or arranging to come back on your own to correct your previous information.

A wrong initial or provisional diagnosis happens around 15 per cent of the time. It could be that there just wasn't the information to make the correct diagnosis, it could be that the patient has a piece of the jigsaw without realizing it, or it could be that the patient has handed over the piece of the jigsaw and the doctor has not realized it or put it in the wrong place. Instead of blaming, work on getting the jigsaw right together. Always ask what else could it be? And how would I know?

Sometimes there is no diagnosis. And even if there is, a diagnosis is only worth having if it improves, or helps you plan your life in some way. Otherwise it's just a label to carry around.

The Right Tests and Investigations

Often, the diagnosis can be made by just listening to you and examining you. If you want to know, it's worth asking your doctor how he or she made the diagnosis and excluded other diagnoses. Hearing your doctor 'think out loud' can help you understand your symptoms, and assess them in future.

The NHS – like all modern health systems – is heavily reliant on diagnostic tests. About 70–80 per cent of all healthcare decisions affecting diagnosis or treatment are influenced by laboratory medicine results, and they play a big part in screening and monitoring – particularly in the management of chronic conditions. Over one-quarter of the population in England, 15.4 million people, have a long-term condition – the number with three or more conditions is expected to increase from 1.9 million in 2008 to 2.9 million in 2018. All those who choose to have their diseases medicalized will have regular tests.

How many of these tests are really needed and actually make a difference to the care you receive is hard to say. As we've seen from the discussion on screening, tests – and the treatments they lead to – have the capacity to cause harm as well as good. How likely a test is to be accurate doesn't just depend on the test result, but also on how likely you are to have the disease in the first place. The lower risk you are, the less likely you are to benefit from any test and the more likely you are to be harmed by a 'false positive' result.

As with any treatment, it's always worth asking, 'How likely am I to benefit from this test?' and 'What is most likely to happen if we did nothing?' All tests have margins or error, and are prone to human error. For a service so crucial to the NHS, pathology receives just 3 per cent of the budget, so labs are under enormous pressure to churn out results quickly.

In general, you should never make a huge decision for or against treatment on the basis of a single test. The NHS should treat you – a whole person – not your test results, and reach a most-likely diagnosis based on all the evidence. If your case is complicated, it's likely to be discussed at a multidisciplinary team meeting, with all the specialists involved in your care, pathologists and other experts offering their opinions. Ask if you can attend, or at least have someone in the team report back to you.

If you want to learn about your tests, their accuracy and the interpretation of the results, ask. You can also ask to have copies of your results – blood tests, scan reports, pathology samples – and copies of the scans too. Keeping your results in date order can help you to spot a trend in results which is often more useful than a single result. If you've had a test and still feel awful, another test – or another opinion with a different investigation – might make a big difference.

As new technology gets ever more sensitive, it picks up more 'false positive' results as well as more real disease. If you have, say, a total body MRI scan, as some private companies are all too willing to offer you, it will almost certainly find shadows, or calcification, or some other 'abnormality' that probably means nothing and can only be resolved by further scanning and investigation – and may never be fully resolved. If you feel well, you can be turned from a happy person into an anxious patient. Doctors call this VOMIT (Victims of Medical Imaging Technology). There's a lot of money to be made from screening, and everyone wants a slice of you when you're well. But you are allowed to say no.

On the other hand, if you feel dreadful, there's likely to be a reason for it. Medicine may not always find it or understand it, but don't be falsely reassured by one single test or group of tests. If symptoms persist, it's worth having investigations or another opinion to see if there are any treatable causes.

Crowdfunding Your Own Care

Britain will forever be remembered as one of the first countries to introduce universal healthcare and one of the last to fund it adequately. We have consistently put less into healthcare than our European neighbours over many decades, despite being the fourth or fifth richest nation in the world. Clearly, we could have afforded more but we chose not to. As in America, an increasing number of UK patients are now having to crowd und private care because the NHS has refused them treatment. One of my neighbours, Georgia 'Porge' Bryant, typified the values of the NHS. When her good friend Abbie got cervical cancer, Porge hosted charity events and helped raise £150,000 for the Teenage Cancer Trust to help other young people affected by cancer.

In September 2017, a year after Abbie lost her fight against cancer, Porge herself was diagnosed with Acute Lymphoblastic Leukaemia (ALL). After 3 months of intense chemotherapy and radiotherapy, and with thanks to the Anthony Nolan Trust for identifying a donor, Porge underwent a bone marrow transplant on January 5, 2018. Following her transplant she spent a gruelling three weeks in isolation as part of her 100 day post-transplant recovery period. Porge responded in text-book fashion to her treatment, improving day by day and showing great courage, humour and resilience. However, just as she was beginning to 'feel sexy' again, her leukaemia returned.

After initially being told that she only had a 'glimmer of hope', the professor in charge of Porge's treatment advised that she was eligible to take part in a clinical trial which has the potential to save her life and help others. This would be funded through research but the drug she needed to keep her alive to enter the trial, Inotuzomab, was not then available on the NHS even though it was widely available in many better funded health services. NICE, the organization that decides what the NHS can afford, initially ruled that although the drug was proven to extend life, its cost was too high. The drug industry too needs to examine its conscience about the prices it charges.

Porge and her family are fighters. Her sister Lottie orchestrated a massive 'gofundme' campaign and raised the required £80,000 from the same local community that had raised funds when Abbie had cancer. Porge started the Inotuzomab and entered the trial. Sadly, treatment was not successful and she died in September 2018. Two days before her death, NICE finally approved Inotuzomab for NHS use.

Porge insisted on being fully-included in decisions about her care and became an expert in understanding her leukaemia. After her death, her family created the Chew Valley Family fund, 'where we will put any left over money from our fundraising to hold for anyone else in the community that may need it in the future, for medical purposes.' As newer and better treatments are developed to treat cancer and other diseases, we will have to pay for them somehow. In an underfunded NHS, crowd-sourcing is becoming more common. The British are unbelievably generous when it comes to giving to those in need, but we would save ourselves a huge amount of harm, hassle and heartache if we simply gave more to health and social care, and made sure it was spent fairly and wisely.

THE RIGHT SUPPORT AFTER DIAGNOSIS

Louise's Story

My mother has dementia. She is not able to be fully involved in all decisions about her care. But if you get to know her, she can be delightful company. The one thing that has transformed her care going into hospital is filling in the 'This Is Me' booklet from the Alzheimer's Society. The more you can tell the staff about a person, the more personalized their care becomes. NHS staff can only know what's important to a person if you tell them. Every patient or carer should fill it in, no matter what they've got.

Nick's Story

The Alzheimer's Society is a godsend. It tells you everything you need to know about the different types of dementia, the symptoms and diagnosis, what it's like living with the disease, what it's like caring for somebody with it, what treatments are available, what research is going on, what help and support is available in your local area if you put your postcode in. It gave us really good advice on advanced care planning so we could make choices and decisions about future care, particularly when my mother is not able to make decisions for herself. There are some really difficult conversations to be had with dementia, but you have to have them and you need to be armed with the correct knowledge to get them right.

Audrey's Story

When I was told I had Parkinson's disease it was like being hit by a

sledgehammer. I didn't take in a word that was said afterwards.
Not a word.

The right diagnosis is clearly important for you to be offered a choice
of treatments that are likely to work. But for a serious, life-changing
diagnosis you need time for it to sink in. You may react with shock,
anger, numbness or denial and not take in anything else other than the
diagnosis. As you come to terms with an illness, you may want to find
out as much as you can about it so you can tackle it head on, or you
may need a slow drip-feed of information and support.

Doctors (especially in hospital) are rightly focused initially on trying
to make the right diagnosis and giving the right immediate treatment,
and put a lot of energy into this. But it's often other members of the
team – nurses, physiotherapists, occupational therapists, speech therapists, clinical psychologists, healthcare assistants – who get you back
on your feet and focused on improving your life. Remember, this is the
purpose of the NHS and yet we often overlook simpler, cheaper ways
of improving patients' lives. Here are two great examples.

Football Therapy

Janette Hynes, an occupational therapist at East London and City Mental Health Trust, had been using football to help patients with severe
mental illness while in hospital, but was disappointed that they had no
team to play with when they got out. Despite resistance from the pre-
vailing attitudes in mainstream football, she set up the Positive Mental
Attitude (PMA) football league in 2002, using her expertise as a professional footballer. When I met Janette, the PMA league had fourteen
teams, with twenty waiting to join, and has resulted in better physical
and mental health for its players. Many have lost the flab, stopped
smoking and got jobs. The league links with social services. Men and
plenty of women love their football and if they don't turn up to training, it's a good predictor of relapse that can be picked up quickly.

What Colour Is My Cancer?

Sue Morgan, a clinical nurse specialist at St James's Hospital, Leeds,
looks after children and teenagers with cancer. One of them asked her,

'What colour is my cancer?' So she set up a service where young patients can view their cancer under a microscope. It's had huge psychological benefits. Many children (and adults) imagine their cancer as a ravenous beast, all hooded, black and menacing, eating away at them. In reality, their cancers looked like 'sausages', 'Granny's wallpaper' and 'jelly beans'. Far from trivializing their illness, it's given the children confidence to fight it. A side effect has been that pathologists have started talking to patients again. This could easily be rolled out across the NHS for peanuts. Or you could be proactive and ask to see your cancer down the microscope. Learn about and know what you're dealing with.

These sorts of simple interventions can be hugely important in helping people cope with illness – and patients are often the best people to support each other. Find out what support groups are available locally and nationally for patients like you.

In an emergency, or when you're given bad news about your health, you may not remember much about what happened and what was said to you, but when you emerge from the brain fog of shock, anger, numbness or denial, you need knowledge and skills quickly, and the courage to use them to get the right care for you (hopefully right first time). This may still happen if you leave all the difficult decisions to the people treating you, but it's more likely to happen if you get as informed and involved in your care as you can. And you're going to need help and support.

I've spoken to many patients, and their carers, who've needed a lot of NHS and social care over the years, usually because they have a life-long illness or disability. And the four things they say that make the biggest difference when it comes to getting the care they need are:

- Finding a good specialist nurse
- Finding a good GP
- Finding a good care worker
- Finding a good charity

If you manage to get access to a specialist nurse, whatever your illness, it can make a huge difference to the quality of your care. They give you knowledge, skills, confidence, courage, kindness and laughter. It's no coincidence that when the NHS has failed badly, often in the care of the most vulnerable or elderly patients, a recurring theme is that there were simply not enough specialist nurses to provide safe care to patients with very complex needs.

Good care workers too are like gold dust. They also give you knowledge, skills, confidence, courage, kindness and laughter – as well as a huge amount of the personal care you can't give to yourself. Every spare penny in the NHS and social care system should be spent on training and employing as many frontline nurses and carers as possible, and making sure all parts of the system are safely staffed. Charities also give you knowledge, skills, confidence, courage, kindness and laughter – and crucially are there to support and advise you if gaps appear in your care, you don't know what you're entitled to or you don't know how to appeal against a decision not to give you what you think you should be entitled to.

Many people facing the challenge of serious illness have a huge thirst for information. Websites can provide many of the facts, but the right specialist nurse can make a huge difference in coming to terms with illness and getting the right care for you. Imagine you've just been told you have multiple sclerosis.

Paul's Story

It is hard to ask questions when you're ill, but it's also essential. If you're stuck with a disease like MS for fifty years, as many people are, you have to coordinate your own care otherwise you just get lost in the system. It's a huge effort and responsibility but if you don't do it, no-one else may. Friends, relatives, charities and health professionals can be incredibly helpful. But ultimately you're the one who has to join up your own care.

I suspected I had something like MS – a reduction in eyesight and colour vision was the first symptom. And I'd looked on the internet, but turned off quickly. Even so, actually getting the diagnosis is still like being hit by a sledgehammer. My consultant was kind, and that really helped, and the nurse was wonderful. They let the diagnosis sink in, just sat with me and then asked if I had any questions. I was in no state to ask anything, so the nurse told my wife and I to think of what we needed to know about the disease and how to cope with it – anything at all – and she'd do her best to answer the questions or find out someone who could.

So I went away and made a list of everything I needed to know. When you move from the land of the well to the land of the ill, life suddenly becomes horribly insecure and uncertain, and the only thing you can cling on to is knowledge. I had a list of fifty-seven questions just to get me up to speed, which I think was more than the nurse was expecting, but she didn't even flinch. She smiled – a kind smile – and we started my education.

It took a few meetings, and she showed me some good websites and chat rooms. The MS Society has been really helpful. But you have to find stuff out for yourself. It takes a long time and some of the answers are scary but it's not as scary as not knowing, and you meet other people through charities and chat rooms who are not just surviving with MS, but living a life.

My original list, which I guess would be similar for anyone with an incurable disease, was massive. I called it the Heinz 57:

1. Why has this happened to me?
2. Why now?
3. Will it kill me?
4. How soon?
5. What exactly is going on in my brain?
6. Have I done anything to bring it on myself?
7. Should I stop smoking?
8. When will people be able to tell that I'm ill?
9. Are there different types of multiple sclerosis?
10. Which type have I got?
11. What stage of the disease am I at?
12. Can I fully recover or have I got it for life?
13. Will I become disabled?
14. Are there any drugs that will reverse the disease or slow it down?
15. What are their side effects?

16. What do I do if I have a flare-up?
17. Will I still be able to work?
18. Do I have to tell my work?
19. What are my rights as an employee?
20. Can I drive?
21. Am I going to pass it on to my children?
22. Do other people in my family need to have tests?
23. Will it make me impotent?
24. Will it make me infertile?
25. Can I have vaccinations?
26. Is it safe to have an anaesthetic?
27. Is there some sort of diet that might help?
28. Should I have oxygen therapy?
29. Should I have vitamin D supplements?
30. Should I avoid dental procedures?
31. Should I have my mercury fillings removed?
32. Is there anything I can do to prevent relapse?
33. Will I go blind?
34. Will I be confined to a wheelchair?
35. Will I be able to speak and swallow?
36. Will my muscles all stiffen up?
37. Will I be in severe pain?
38. Will I lose sensation?
39. Will I become incontinent?
40. Will I need a catheter?
41. Where will the money come from when I'm ill?
42. Is there any financial assistance available now?
43. Will I be able to look after my children?
44. Will my wife leave me?
45. Will I get depressed?
46. Are you absolutely sure it's multiple sclerosis?
47. Why?
48. Could it be anything else?
49. Will I have a horrible death, confined to bed, totally dependent, incontinent, unable to speak eat or swallow?
50. Will I get pressure sores?

51. Shall I make a will?

52. Shall I make an advanced directive?

53. Should I give my wife power of attorney or wait and see how she takes it?

54. How close are we to a cure?

55. Are there any trials of new drugs I could enter?

56. If I start looking for information online, will it just really depress and frightened me?

57. Who can I trust to answer all these questions honestly, kindly and accurately?

There's a huge amount to learn if you want to get on top of an illness like MS, but if you stick at it, you can soon know as much as your GP about some things and even more about others. There's so much to take on board that I didn't even consider at first that I might not be getting the drugs I needed until my (wonderful) nurse said she thought I should be on a disease-modifying drug. The consultant thought so too, but the NHS wasn't funding it in my area, even though you could get it in other parts of the UK, and he thought it would be kinder not to tell me. You assume the NHS automatically gives you the treatment you need wherever you happen to live in the UK. The idea of a postcode lottery, and having to fight for drugs that other people are given automatically, is a bit dispiriting. But you have to do it.

Paul, thirty-two, teacher

I'm a patron, adviser or supporter to nine charities, and the reason I find it hard to turn them down is that I keep meeting patients and carers who were drowning in the NHS and were rescued by a charity. It's another overriding message of this book that if you need a crash course in surviving and thriving with your illness, or how to negotiate the complexity, unfairness and variable standards of care that exist in all health systems, you need to find the right nurse and the right charity. There is no guarantee of success, but if you don't manage to get the right care, right first time, they are often in the strongest position to support you in your fight for it. Your GP and consultant team are crucial too, but the extra advocacy of a charity and the wisdom and kindness of a great nurse can make all the difference.

When you get a new diagnosis, you don't know what you don't know. Figuring out what questions you want to ask, and which ones take priority, is key. Time is so tight in the NHS, you rarely have time for more than three questions in a consultation. Paul had fifty-seven. Question fifty-seven, at the bottom of his list, is one of the most important: 'Who can I trust to answer all these questions honestly, kindly and accurately?'

A lot of charities and patient groups receive money from drug companies because they don't get enough public donations to keep them alive, and drug companies are obviously keen to work with patients to share expertise and raise awareness of what they're hoping to sell to the NHS. Funding sources should be publicly declared on their website but even when they are, the accusation will always be that health charities end up doing lobbying on behalf of drug companies. Fortunately, we have NICE (the National Institute of Health and Care Excellence) which tries to strip away the bias and get to the truth of how effective a new drug is and whether the NHS can afford it.

I'm a big fan of NICE, although it's far from perfect and should be challenged, and I hold the same views about the NHS, the drug industry and charities. All are largely forces for good but they're run by humans so there will inevitably be some pockets of very poor or corrupt practice that need to be exposed. When a charity is very hostile to NICE, I get suspicious. When it assertively challenges a decision on behalf of patients, while acknowledging that money is limited, hard decisions have to be made and drug companies should consider charging less for their products, I say good for you.

A bigger role for charities is making sure everyone gets the treatments NICE says they should be getting by law (it approves far more drugs and new technologies than it turns down) and that all NHS care is delivered to the proper standard that NICE also determines. If we just focused relentlessly on improving the quality of care for the drugs and treatments we should be using already, it would lead to huge improvements in the NHS. Which is why you, as a patient, need to know all the treatment options available to you.

For example, in May 2014, NICE approved a drug called Alemtuzumab as an option for treating adults with a type of multiple sclerosis called 'active relapsing–remitting'. It's already used to treat chronic lymphocytic leukaemia. Indeed leukaemia treatment, like HIV treatment, is an area where the drug advances have been stunningly good, but the NHS needs to be able to afford the drugs.

Alemtuzumab is an antibody that binds to cells of the immune system (B and T cells), causing their destruction and stopping them attacking the brain and spinal cord. It has some serious side effects but can be very effective in slowing down the progress of the disease. Some patients even appear to recover partially from their disability. Here's the rub. It costs £56,360 for the full course of treatment, plus the money needed to give the drug and do regular blood and safety checks. NICE – after very detailed deliberations – has judged it to work well enough to justify the cost, and all NHS patients whose doctor thinks they should be getting it and who consent to trying it, should now – by law in England – be getting it (within three months of the NICE judgement).

However, different parts of the NHS are in different financial situations and may have different priorities, and you may need a charity on your side to campaign on your behalf. The MS Society offers very clear guidance on how to appeal if you are denied a drug your doctor thinks will benefit you and you wish to take. It differs in all four countries, but the guidance can be applied to any drug or technology, and is very detailed. You may not succeed, but using the expertise of a well-recognized charity gives you your best chance of success.

Approximately 100,000 people in the UK have multiple sclerosis. A 2013 report from the MS Society found that only 40 per cent of eligible people with MS in the UK are currently on disease-modifying drugs. This report on MS treatment and care ranked the UK twenty-fifth out of twenty-seven comparator countries with regard to MS drugs. Across Europe, only Poland and Romania fare worse. Access to treatments varies geographically; MS patients in Northern Ireland are more than twice as likely to be taking a DMT (disease-modifying therapy) than those in Wales.

Knowing what treatment you're entitled to in the NHS is no guarantee you'll get it, but it gives you more of a chance than not knowing. If you're not getting a DMT and you think you're entitled, ask why not and contact the MS Society. As Paul put it: 'I'm getting the right drugs partly because I'm lucky to live where I do, but also I think because I learned what care I was entitled to, got my consultant's agreement, had the support of a great nurse, GP and charity, and we kept asking.'

Don't be shy about asking for what you're entitled to.

Using Charities to Correct False Assumptions

As well as giving you the right information and support, charities can be enormously helpful in correcting wrong information or assumptions that may follow the correct diagnosis and drug treatment. Sexually transmitted infections are more properly called sexually shared infections. We share pleasure and, if we don't use condoms (and sometimes even when we do), we share bugs. Very rarely does anyone pass on an infection on purpose. Many people with sexually shared infections have no symptoms at all, and are completely unaware that they are passing them on. It's also really important to understand that some infections, such as warts and herpes, can be carried for many years without knowing, and a flare-up at any stage in a relationship does not mean infidelity. Often the psychological and relationship damage caused by ignorance about these infections is far more harmful than the infections themselves. And once again, compassionate and wise charity helpliners can direct you to the right NHS care.

'EIGHTY PER CENT OF PEOPLE WITH HERPES DON'T KNOW IT'

Linda's Story

My herpes story is typical in many ways but not in others. I want people to know how a common and unimportant, but stigmatized virus, almost destroyed my marriage. I hope that my story will help others to avoid the trap I nearly fell into. My name is not Linda. My husband is not called Geoff. Unlike Embarrassing Bodies volunteers, we're not quite brave enough to be completely 'out' of the herpes closet. What I can say is that the man who gave me herpes is the most wonderful, considerate, supportive person I have ever met. And if you get the right information, kindly given, living with herpes isn't nearly as scary as it's hyped up to be.

When I was twenty-nine, I was introduced by a friend to Geoff. We connected immediately. He was kind, wise and funny. After a few dates, it was clear that we were well matched. We talked openly of previous partners, and decided to take our time, be responsible and have check-ups before we had sex. We went on a 'date' to a sexual health clinic, were given the all clear, praised for our responsible attitude and started a very happy life with lots of sex. In six months we had moved in together, a year after that we were married.

Two days into our honeymoon in Bali, I thought I had thrush. I'd always been prone to it, but had learned to live with it and I knew how to treat it. This time it seemed slightly different – sorer and more insistent. I went to the bathroom, pulled out my vanity mirror and had a look. I could see the beginning of what looked like blisters. This wasn't right. What was it? Where had it come from? – Geoff, I presumed – but what could I do about it in Indonesia?

I was in a state of shock. I mumbled to Geoff that I felt queasy and needed a doctor. I tracked down the travel company host. He gave me a card and sketched out directions on the back of it. I grabbed Geoff and ten minutes later, we were sitting in a waiting room. I went in on my own. The doctor examined me and just said, 'Herpes'. I can remember feeling repulsed and sick. When I was at college, a friend was diagnosed with herpes. The trauma had kept us awake for weeks, but I thought she was a drama queen and hadn't been very sympathetic. I started to wish I had been. I was given a pack of antiviral tablets and then I was back in the waiting room staring at Geoff in disbelief. He knew something was up but I bottled it up until we were back in the hotel room. At thirty-one, I was thinking

of having a baby, maybe even conceived on honeymoon. There are lots of things you wish for on your honeymoon. Herpes isn't one of them.

He was uncomprehending and bewildered. My mind kept going back to his stag night. Who knows what went on? Maybe even before that. I made my mind up to divorce him as soon as we got back home. I knew we were clear of infections when we met so I had proof that he had been shagging around. The rest of the honeymoon was spent in silence. I was sore and feverish. I stayed in the room half the time sobbing. Geoff wandered around like a lost puppy, trying to placate me. 'It's not me,' he kept saying. 'This is all a mistake.'

This just made me really mad. After giving me herpes, the least he could do was fess up and be honest about what he had been up to. My resolve to divorce him hardened.

By the time we returned my symptoms were on the mend. Back home we barely acknowledged each other and I called my sister for support. This was my first stroke of luck. I had looked on the internet but she found the website of the Herpes Viruses Association. The information on their website was in stark contrast to what I had read elsewhere. 'Common.' 'Usually undiagnosed.' 'Eighty per cent who have it do not know.' These were staggering statements. How could all these people damn well not know? It was agony. I could barely go to the toilet when it started.

Two days later I plucked up courage and phoned the helpline, still in a bit of an emotional state. The helpliner was calm, sympathetic and surprisingly helpful. He filled in the gaps in my knowledge and suggested that I attend an NHS sexual health clinic to get the diagnosis confirmed and to make quite sure there weren't any other infections. I told him that we'd done that at the beginning of our relationship and were given the all clear. He explained that herpes is not tested for when you have a check-up – unless the doctor sees symptoms. And many people get such mild symptoms they don't know they have it.

The NHS clinic was brilliant. They explained that they couldn't confirm the herpes as the symptoms had almost gone, but the health adviser, Leonie, confirmed what the Herpes Viruses Association had said and handed me a copy of their Guide. I remembered her name, as she was the first person I met face to face who really convinced me that having herpes is normal. Most people who've had sex have at some stage shared herpes viruses and the HPV viruses that can cause warts and cervical cancer. Usually they don't cause symptoms, but the infections themselves are so common as to be normal, and may have happened years previously. Often, the fear and blame surrounding infection does far more damage than the viruses themselves.

That was when my certainty about Geoff's infidelity began to crumble. I was completely floored. He may have been unfaithful but it was far more likely that he'd had it since before we met and not realized. This knowledge changed my world. By this time he had moved out and was kipping on a friend's floor. The atmosphere had become too much for him. I sent him a text: 'We need to meet and talk.' That evening he came round and the whole saga began to make sense for both of us. We worked out that it had all come from a pimple – and he had been getting this pimple, near the base of his penis, for years. 'It's nothing. It's hardly ever there. I had no idea.'

There is one thing you can say about Geoff, he doesn't hold a grudge. I know he was the source of our herpes, but it was hardly his fault and I had given him a hell of a time over it. Five years later, and we're just about able to laugh at it. I do get occasional recurrences. Geoff still gets the 'pimple', we have unprotected sex whenever we feel like it because we've already shared whatever it is we have to share. Quite honestly, my thrush is still the bigger problem. Herpes has gone from being a marriage breaker to a minor irritation with the right knowledge, sensitive reassurance and the test of time. Oh, and I had twins by natural childbirth. Another herpes myth bites the dust.

Myths about any illness are intensely damaging. Embarrassing Bodies and Embarrassing Problems are two wonderful websites to bust myths and get the right care. The Herpes Viruses Association will set you straight about herpes. Sexual health clinics are open access (you don't need to go to your GP first), you can phone up or turn up to most and you are entirely in control of who knows what. Nobody will tell your parents or GP if you don't want them to. Many deal with sexual problems, rape and assault, pregnancy testing and contraception too, all under one roof.

THE RIGHT DECISION FOR YOU

If you've decided to use the NHS, you then have to decide whether you want to act on the advice you've been given. Only half of patients take their prescribed drugs properly (i.e. in order for them to work) and for life-long prescriptions it may be as low as one in three. You don't have to do anything a doctor says, and you may have good reasons for not doing so, but to keep cashing in prescriptions and not taking them is a huge waste of NHS resources. If you've weighed up the risks and don't want to take the treatment, or you're getting side effects, tell your doctor. We'd far rather hear the truth than think the drugs just aren't working.

If you've thought about your needs and your goals in advance of your consultation, and your doctor or nurse agrees, you can then move on to how likely any treatment is to help you achieve them. If you share in decisions about your care, you're likely to get better care that's right for you. To make a good choice, you must let your doctor know your hopes and fears, what matters most to you in your life and what you must avoid. You also need to know the risks, benefits and likely success rates of the possible treatments. And it's always worth asking, 'What if we did nothing?' The body has evolved an extraordinary capacity to heal itself in time.

At the end of every consultation, check:

- What is my main problem?

- What do I need to do now?

- Why is it important for me to do this?

- What if it doesn't get better?

A lot of decisions don't need to be made there and then, and if you're committing yourself to surgery or drugs for life, it's worth taking time over that decision and not rushing it in a consultation.

The kind of questions you need to ask yourself are:

- What are my options?

- What are the pros and cons of each option for me?

- How do I get support to help me make a decision that is right for me?

- What is likely to happen if we did nothing?

There are shared decision aids for many medical choices these days that guide you through your options (http://sdm.rightcare.nhs.uk/), mobile apps and a great general aid from Ottawa for making any difficult decision in life and healthcare (https://decisionaid.ohri.ca/). You can then go back to your GP with any questions. The evidence is clear that patients who share in decisions with their doctors and nurses usually make better choices, feel better and get better. But you've got to find a doctor who wants to share with you and has time to do it. Or you could just ask, 'What would you do doctor?'

How to Make Better Decisions

Your attitude to risk and which ones you are happy taking depends on your values and life experiences. If a close relative or friend has had cancer, it might tip you towards taking a daily aspirin; if they've had a big stomach bleed it might steer you away. The trouble with taking any drug for prevention is that you never really know if it's worked, whereas you tend to notice serious side effects. In an ideal world, you'd have time to share all these tricky decisions with a health professional who has the time and expertise to guide you through the decision-making process. And there's good evidence that this 'shared decision-making' leads to better choices, better health and better healthcare.

However, to succeed, there needs to be enough time for patients and professionals to understand what is important to the other person when choosing a treatment. Time is a rarity in the NHS, but fortunately most decisions don't need to be made there and then, so you can take your time until you feel comfortable that a decision is right for you. And remember it's always worth researching 'What is most likely to happen if I did nothing?'

The stages of shared decision-making with, say, a doctor are:

- Your doctor gives you information about all the treatment options for your health problem, and whether any particular option is medically better for you based on his or her understanding of your personal medical history and test results.

- You give information about your life and experiences of illness and treatment, and which option might fit better with your life and what matters most to you. It might be different from the 'medically best' treatment.

- You have a conversation, listen to and understand each other's point of view and agree the reasons why the treatment chosen is the best one for you. You have the final vote if you want to.

Decisions about treatment are getting ever more complicated as technology advances and more options are available. The choices can feel overwhelming. One way of coping with this is to break the decision down into manageable chunks.

- The first chunk might be 'What is most likely to happen if we did nothing?'

- If you decide that doing nothing is not the best option, and the benefits of treatment are worth pursuing, ask, 'In what ways am I likely to benefit?' Remember, you don't just want to get out of hospital alive, you want all the hassle of treatment to lead to an improvement in the quality of your life. Where is the evidence it will do this?

- Finally you can chunk the treatment options into different categories. You might choose between drug therapy, radiotherapy or surgery for example. Choose the category or combination that's right for you before exploring it in more detail.

- Remember newer is not always better, and neither is more. The best and safest option is often a) the tried-and-tested one that we know works, and b) the minimal intervention needed to do the job.

- If you choose an option that requires technical skill, rather than just swallowing tablets, you may then want to explore where the centres of excellence are, what their comparative results are and whether you are entitled to be treated there.

- Centres of excellence often do high-quality research and are linked to reputable charities. Once you've tracked down the charities, they can give you invaluable information about where to go to get the right care for you.

THE RIGHT DRUG TREATMENT FOR YOU

How Many Drugs Do I Need?

Giving drugs is what doctors do. It's by far the most common form of medical intervention. Four out of five people aged over seventy-five years take a prescription drug and 36 per cent are taking four or more. Patients don't like taking drugs, or struggle to take so many, and so up to 50 per cent of drugs are not taken as prescribed – which is a huge waste of time, effort and money (estimated to be £300 million a year) that could be spent on more nurses.

Adverse reactions to medicines are a major factor in 5–17 per cent of hospital admissions. The more drugs you take, the more likely you are to have side effects, and if you've been admitted already because of a side effect you're more likely to be admitted again with another side effect. Many people admitted due to drug side effects are gaining very little benefit from the drug. Why has this madness been allowed to happen and can it be stopped?

Doctors are encouraged, even incentivized, to prescribe drugs to reduce the risk of something nasty happening to you such as a stroke, heart attack or kidney failure. There are often very clear guidelines to prevent or treat an individual disease, and when to start drugs – often for life. You collect diseases or risk factors as you get older, more guidelines kick in and you end up on more drugs unless you opt out. You may end up on lots of drugs, each giving you a smallish benefit in reducing your risk of a disease, but all lumped together sometimes they make you feel unwell and increase your risk of a hospital admission. Overall, they may not make you live longer at all, and may well not help you live more happily.

Weighing Up the Risks and Benefits of a Drug

One way is to suck it and see. If you feel fine on your statin, and your doctor thinks it's a good idea to reduce your cholesterol, that may be good enough for you. You're the one who takes the drug, you're the one who's best placed to spot side effects. Speak up if you think you have.

Generally, you should take as few drugs as possible, and at the lowest dose that works. The bottom line with drugs (indeed any treatment) is that newer is not always better and more is not always better. In the case of the older patient, less is often more.

The trustworthy website RxISK has come up with questions you should ask about any drug offered to you that could save your life: http://wp.rxisk.org/know-your-rx-drug-rxisk/.

- How does this drug work, how much improvement can I expect, and how soon?

- If I don't take this drug now, and instead wait for a while, what will happen?

- What are the most likely side effects?

- Are there any rare serious side effects?

- Are there any permanent problems this drug can cause?

- If this is a new drug, why can't I take an older drug?

- Can I try a lower dose?

- What date will we review my use/dose of this drug?

- Are there problems stopping the drug or any special considerations on stopping or changing dose that I should watch for?

- Are there any potential interactions with food, my other medical conditions, or my current medications?

- Might this drug affect my weight/sleep/hair/skin/nails/mood/sex life and/or relationships, and if so, how?

- Do I need to stop this drug before I get pregnant?

These questions are all reasonable to me but it's hard to get through them all in a ten-minute consultation, so you may need several goes. We can all turn to jelly when faced with a doctor, and rarely do we remember anything other than the diagnosis. I'm a great fan of lists.

Not just for taking into the consultation, but for making during the consultation and even for leaving with the doctor to remind them what they have promised to do for you.

Time is always of the essence in a consultation and you can never cover all the bases or all the points on your list. So if you are, say, on a medication and want to know more about it, I would pay a visit to the website http://wp.rxisk.org. RxISK says it's the first free, independent website where patients, doctors and pharmacists can research prescription drugs and easily report a drug side effect. It helps users spot drug side effects and it'll make people a lot more sceptical about the claims made by drug companies.

Medicine relies on trust and there's a danger that if you stop taking a drug because you can't be sure the drug company isn't hiding the results that show it doesn't work or has unpleasant side effects, you could do yourself some harm. But like the NHS, there's an unpleasant tendency for harm and errors to be covered up in the drug industry rather than owned up to and acted on. Informed, earned trust is a much safer mind-set that blindly believing that a drug is safe or right for you just because the government allowed it, the regulators approved it, your doctor prescribed it and your pharmacist dispensed it. When you're given a new drug, you could ask, 'Are all trials about this drug in the public domain?' and 'How do you know?' (An ethical drug company will have signed up to www.alltrials.net.) I've researched my two blood pressure drugs (Ramapril and Amlodipine). I think they're safe, I don't get any side effects, my blood pressure's come down a treat and I've cut my risk of having a stroke or heart attack on stage, the ultimate horror for any comedian (not least because the audience would just sit there and assume it was part of the act).

If you like numbers, there is another way of assessing if a drug is worth taking:

- Ask about 'numbers needed to treat' and 'numbers needed to harm'.

- The 'number needed to treat' (NNT) is the average number of patients who require to be treated for one to benefit. You might also want to know what the benefit you're aiming for is (e.g. avoiding

death, a flare-up of your arthritis, a heart attack, a stroke or a verte-
bral fracture). You also want to know over what period the benefit
accrues. If you have to take a drug for ten years to get a small benefit, you're far better off buying a dog (I have two).

- 'Number needed to harm' (NNH) is the average number of people
  exposed to a medication for one person to suffer an adverse event
  (death, bleeding from the gut, kidney failure, falling over in the pot-
  ting shed, etc).

- The reason I like NNT and NNH is that most of us understand the
  difference in likely benefit between a one in ten drug or a one in a
  hundred drug. There are lots of other ways of 'spinning' risk to put
  you in favour of, or against, a treatment. For example, say you've
  had a heart attack or suffer from angina and you want to reduce your
  risk of dying from heart disease. A doctor might say, 'I think a cho-
  lesterol-lowering drug is a good thing,' and leave it at that. But if you
  asked how likely the treatment was to help you, in numerical terms,
  there are lots of ways the information could be phrased:

  - 'If you take this drug every day for five years, your relative risk
    of death will be reduced by nearly 40 per cent.'

  - 'If you take this drug every day for five years, your risk of death
    will fall from 8 per cent to 5 per cent.'

  - 'If thirty-three people like you take this drug every day for five
    years, one death will be prevented but I don't know whether it
    will be yours.'

  - 'If you swallowed 1,825 tablets of this drug at a rate of one a day
    for five years and at a prescription cost of £426, your absolute
    risk of death would fall by 0.9%. The recognized side effects are
    muscle damage, headache, abdominal pain, nausea, vomiting,
    hair loss, anaemia, dizziness, depression, nerve damage, hepa-
    titis, jaundice, pancreatitis and hypersensitivity syndrome.'

Which of the statements is most likely to convince you to take the drug? In fact, all the statements are about the same statin but the first – the relative risk reduction – is the one most quoted in press releases, advertisements and newspaper headlines. Naturally, the drug companies are keen to hype the benefits, and doctors may put a positive slant on prescribing some drugs because we get paid to hit targets. Asking for the absolute, as well as the relative, risk reduction is a good way of getting the benefits of a treatment in perspective. But I find NNT and NNH easier (although they're only estimates – ultimately what works is what works for you).

DRUG WARNING: Elderly patients are at high risk of confusion and falls caused by medication, but the drug trials are never done on elderly patients so the published NNH is likely to be higher than the real values. Also, we don't know how to accurately add up all the possible harms for all the drugs you're taking. But we can ask you how all the drugs are making you feel. And often you (like me) will feel fine on your drugs.

We used to dose a lot of people up to the eyeballs with diazepam (Valium) to help them sleep at night, but we've largely stopped doing it because the NNT is thirteen but the NNH is six. It's also more addictive than heroin. However, some patients found it incredibly helpful for them and were very distressed when their doctors stopped prescribing it. Large trials guide the NHS into deciding what treatments it should be paying for, but these trials are full of imperfections and only you can tell us if a treatment does, or doesn't, work for you and what it's side effects are when *you* take it.

How to Take Drugs Safely

Learning From an Expert
Some drugs may give you huge improvements, in which case stick with them and learn to respect them. A drug that has amazing effects is often coloured by side effects and has to be handled with care. This can take a bit of effort but if you're up to it, it's worth it. I was recently sent these top tips for avoiding adverse drug events for patients with chronic diseases. It was written by Kelly Young, aka Rheumatoid Arthritis Warrior, who is one of the most inspirational patient leaders and advocates I have encountered. If you want a quick dose of knowledge,

skills, confidence and courage as a patient living with any chronic disease, check out her site. It can lead you to a whole community of 'e-patients' sharing their inspiration, humour and expertise. They are confident, welcoming and encouraging, and it could well rub off on you. Check out e-Patient Dave (www.epatientdave.com) too. You will see why and how patient power is the future of health systems across the world.

The goals for Kelly's website are:

- Help patients find information and encouragement so they can live the best life possible.

- Increase awareness about rheumatoid arthritis and correct common misconceptions.

- Present the patient story in a way that may increase understanding of the disease by doctors and researchers.

Although she's writing in America, I was struck by how spot-on her medication safety tips were for the NHS.

Twenty Essential Medication Safety Tips

1. Use a single pharmacy as much as possible. As an important safety partner, your regular pharmacist can help prevent dangerous errors such as overlapping prescription ingredients or medication interaction problems.

2. Use a medication safe to lock up controlled substances or medicines that might be a danger to others or a target for theft.

3. Make sure your doctor has an updated list of everything you take, including over-the-counter (OTC) supplements and herbal medications. Share this information with your pharmacist when you ask his or her advice.

4. Carry medications in carefully labelled containers, preferably in original containers. A pharmacist can provide a small duplicate bottle if you need to carry only part of a prescription.

5. Keep a log of doses taken or count out doses for each day of the week or time of day and place in labelled pill containers.

6. Look over package information leaflets and store in a file for future reference. If you misplace one, they can usually be found in PDF form by searching online.

7. Teach young children to respect medication as something that can be helpful, but dangerous if not used properly, like cars and stovetops.

8. Dispose of old medications carefully, asking a pharmacist if you are unsure of the safest way to discard. Do not flush medications down the toilet.

9. Pay attention to whether medicines should be taken before or after eating or whether there are foods that should be avoided with your medication because they could increase or decrease absorption. Your pharmacist should be able to help you with this.

10. Pay attention to the maximum daily dosage and the optimal dosing schedule, especially in light of other medications.

11. Know what the active ingredients are in a medicine so you can be aware of proper dosing or which medications contain the same ingredient or same type of ingredient.

12. Know what a medication is for and what to expect. Whenever a new medicine is prescribed, ask, 'How will this help me?' 'How will I know if it's working?'

13. Know what side effects to expect and which ones are routine versus serious signs. With new medications, ask your doctor and pharmacist: 'What things do I need to watch out for?'

14. Check medications when picking them up at the pharmacy or when they arrive in the mail. Make sure they are the dose and brand you expect.

15. Never assume dosing with a different bottle. Medications can vary in strength by brand or when labelled for different age or usage, so always check labelled dosage even with a familiar medicine.

16. Call your doctor or pharmacist with any side effects that seem different or more severe than you expected. Sometimes the dose can be adjusted, but it also guards against possible error in dosage, allergy, or a drug interaction.

17. If you develop an acute illness or infection, ask your doctor whether to suspend or alter your routine disease treatments. It's a good idea to ask ahead of time because you might need to know on a Saturday night.

18. Avoid sharing. It is not safe to share prescriptions with others who have not been prescribed that medication.

19. Do not skip regular blood tests related to your medications. This is a crucial part of the medication regimen, and changes can be detected early with regular testing.

20. Know whether your medication can be stopped suddenly or whether the dose must be reduced gradually.

This is excellent advice, particularly if you're on lots of pills that you've decided you probably should take and you need to be closely monitored. But are you interested, engaged and confident enough to want to take such responsibility and control over your disease management? At the very least, simply carry a list of your drugs, what they're for, who prescribed them and how long for. It's vital information if you're suddenly taken ill. The only drug I carry around with me is aspirin – in my wallet – in case I or someone with me has a heart attack. It can dramatically reduce the damage to your heart muscle.

THE RIGHT OPERATION AND SPECIALIST FOR YOU

One of the most unsettling things about all modern health services is that standards and practices vary a lot. This is true across the board, from general practice to super specialist care. Some of that variation is unavoidable. By chance alone, in any time period, half of all doctors or hospitals will be below average even if they were equally good. Doctors and hospitals who treat poorer and sicker patients will have higher death rates than those that don't. League tables can be very hard to interpret fairly.

For surgery, the decisions you face can be more complicated because the evidence for what operations work (i.e. are likely to improve the quality of your life in the long term) is less convincing than for drugs, which are more easily (though still imperfectly) tested by randomized controlled trials. So often you're led by the experience, opinion and ability of the surgeon in front of you, which may be very different to the experience, opinion and ability of the surgeon next door, or down the road, or in a specialist centre several hundred miles away.

Choosing the Right Care After a Wrong Diagnosis

- A serious diagnosis can be wrong.

- There is always more than one treatment option.

- The choice that's right for you may not be right for others, nor what a doctor recommends.

- Specialists may only suggest the treatments they themselves can do.

- Do your research to find the right option for you.

- Getting another opinion can make a huge difference.

Healthcare can sometimes present very complex ethical choices, and sometimes the treatment choices offered to you will be limited by what's available in a particular hospital rather than what's available in the wider NHS. It can take good fortune, research and persistence to get the care that's right for you.

'FOR THREE DAYS I LIVED WITH THE HORROR OF A CANCER DIAGNOSIS, BUT I DIDN'T HAVE CANCER AT ALL'

Helen's Story

My story begins with my six paternal aunts. Five had breast cancer, three terminally. The sixth and youngest aunt decided to have preventative mastectomies after seeing her sisters' fates twenty-five years ago . . . the first Angelina Jolie! As I grew up I remember always feeling that it would get me one day and I completely 'got' my aunt's decision, despite the vast majority of people thinking she was mad. To me it made utter sense.

In my thirties I met a scientist from Cancer Research UK. He listened to my aunts' stories and asked if I was being looked after in an NHS family breast clinic. I didn't know they existed but went off to my GP for a referral. My GP didn't know they existed either but was happy to investigate and sure enough I was referred to my local hospital which had one. It was a year before I was seen and I was then referred on to Guy's Hospital genetic team. They took down loads of information and took bloods from my only surviving aunt who had had breast cancer. We were found not to have the known BRCA gene mutations but told that we would almost certainly have a genetic mutation, it was just one that hadn't been discovered yet!

I then was advised to have annual mammograms until I became of the age that I got them anyway under the national screening programme. A year later, just before my next mammogram (June 2011, aged thirty-eight), I dreamt I had a breast lump. The next morning I was so perturbed by my dream I did a breast exam, and sure enough I had a lump. It was hard to find as it was against my ribs but there it was.

I went to my local breast one-stop clinic four days later and was seen by the consultant. She examined me, was amazed I'd found the lump and gave me a score of 4/5 and sent me for a mammogram which I had there and then. They had to take several, as the lump was so close to my ribs (ouch!), and that also gave me a 4/5 score and I was sent round the corridor for an ultrasound and biopsy.

The ultrasound gave me a 5/5 score and I was sent back to the surgeon, this time with the breast support nurse (by then her presence meant I knew this was bad news!). They believed I had a grade three invasive tumour, at which point my premonition had come true, I was going to be like my aunts, and my world felt like it was going to fall apart. They recommended double mastectomies due to my family history and that it would be done the following week. In the meantime I was to go home, and return in three days for biopsy results.

For three days I lived with the horror of a cancer diagnosis. I told my family, my three children, some friends. When I went in to see the consultant again she was wreathed in smiles, they couldn't believe they were wrong, I didn't have breast cancer after all, it was a fibroadenoma. They rechecked my biopsy to be sure. Everyone was so pleased but I felt I had been slapped in the face, it was like I'd been caught drink driving and managed to get away without a ban. I never felt the joy everyone else was experiencing. However, I knew immediately I was never going to live through a cancer diagnosis again if I could help it.

I saw the consultant again who said she thought it would be very sensible for me to have preventative mastectomies; if it were her, she would. She said it would be available on the NHS and that as a breast oncoplastic surgeon she would do it. She said I had to have a 'lat dorsi' reconstruction, would remove my nipples and that she would do one breast first and then bring me back six months later to do the other side and then back later again for nipple reconstruction and tattooing. By then I'd done some research online and through friends, and I knew I wanted them doing together, one big hit! I also said I wanted nipple sparing procedure as research was proving this to be a viable option with minimal risk. She said no. It was basically her way only. I felt completely backed into a corner.

At the same time this was going on I had been referred to a plastic surgeon for a mole removal. As he was removing it, I spoke to him about breast reconstructions and my experience. He told me that I should see a colleague of his at East Grinstead hospital, Europe's largest breast reconstruction and plastic surgery hospital. I then met Mr Martin Jones, the consultant of my dreams. He advised me to have a breast surgeon do my mastectomies and that at the same time he would reconstruct my breasts. He informed me of many ways it could be done. Using abdominal muscle transfers, chest wall muscle flaps, inner thigh transfer, a flap from my bottom even, all with or without nipples.

I had choice. He wrote copious notes, made drawings, and photocopied them all for my husband and I to mull over. We met three times over a few months and decided on 'serratus/pec muscle flap', nipple sparing, all in one hit surgery. He has been the most excellent surgeon I have ever met, his time, his compassion, his understanding and his humour have all been superb. I had my surgery in June 2012, initially with Carry On film expander implants, quite surreal watching someone inflate your boobs on a weekly basis! In October 2012 I had these exchanged for permanent silicone implants, like putting on slippers after you've been wearing stilettos all day! My path report showed I had precancerous changes, so I really did beat the bitch that is cancer.

So what did I learn from this? I am now so pro-choice. My initial consultant was lovely, very sympathetic and caring but as a patient you are restricted by your consultant's abilities. I did my research and I knew I could go elsewhere and that there were alternative treatments, so I opted for another opinion. So many others don't know this is an option or don't know that their treatment could be done by other means. There are often other options but you may not be told about them and you need both the will and means to search, and some good fortune from chance conversations, to track them down.

I also think specialists should accept their potential limitations. My first surgeon would have been ideal if I'd had breast cancer and radiotherapy before surgery. She should've been magnanimous enough to say, actually, in your position you should see Mr X as he can perform far more different types of reconstructions for a person in your situation.

Learning From Helen

If you were in Helen's situation, would you be as brave as her? Would you do the research, find out that you were entitled to go elsewhere and actually do it? Or are you happy to accept the care offered locally to you to support your local NHS? You need to question yourself before you can decide what questions you want to ask the people treating you. In 1996, after the first series of *Trust Me, I'm a Doctor* on BBC2, I suggested a list of questions you might want to ask any person treating you for a serious life-threatening or life-limiting disease. The suggestion was largely dismissed as something British patients didn't want to do or weren't capable of doing. Twenty years later, some patients are bravely asking questions and getting proper informed consent for their specialist treatment.

- Are you a specialist for this condition?

- What are my options?

- What are the pros and cons of each option for me?

- How do I get support to help me make a decision that is right for me?

- What are your personal (or your team's) outcome figures for each of these options?

- How do they compare with the NHS average?

- Do you know of any other specialist team in the NHS who has more expertise than you or who can offer me options you are not able to?

In an emergency, you won't have a choice but NHS emergency care is often excellent. For most other treatment you don't have to decide on the spur of the moment, and it's worth taking time to think, reflect on what you've been told and do some research online if you can. Specialist NHS centres for most conditions don't hide the fact and often do a lot of the research too, which is another way of tracking them down. The NHS website can help. But by far the quickest way of wising up when you really need to is to tap into the expertise and support of a good charity.

How Do You Find the Right Specialist?

- Not all consultants will be specialists for your condition.

- You should be given clear information about their results and expertise.

- Getting the right specialist may be the most important decision you ever make.

Surgeons are often the ones who hit the headlines when NHS care goes wrong, because their results are very immediate and hard to hide. But variable standards of care occur in every health system and in every specialty. Having your diabetes or asthma poorly managed in general practice can be as life-threatening as major surgery. The question is, how much are you willing or able to improve your own care, check out the care you should be getting, check that care you are getting is the right standard and speak up or go elsewhere if it's not. Often, we just go with the flow of what our doctor recommends. But as we learned from Helen, your GP may not be in the loop, you may have to do your own research, and finding the right specialist can be the most important choice you ever make. Even more so when it's for your children.

Feedback from a Parent on the NHS Website

My son had several surgeries for hypospadius (where the hole in the penis is on the underside, not the end) as a baby through the urology team at my local hospital. He has wet the bed constantly since then, now aged thirteen. They kept bringing him back in for procedures to try and open the end where he had the surgery which they said was too tight, but just at the tip. They also kept prescribing lots of different drugs resulting in him being off sick from school because they made him very ill, and they kept telling me the bedwetting was unrelated to the surgery. In desperation this year I got my son referred to UCLH instead and they have had to reverse more or less all of the surgery done locally, they said it would definitely be affecting the bedwetting because the previous surgery had caused such a narrowing and not just at the tip. Already we are seeing a difference. I am so disappointed, this should have been picked up years ago, he has missed school trips and sleepovers and I was made to feel like a mother who was imagining things. A ten-minute chat with a consultant every six months was not good enough, the urology team should have paid more attention and been more interested.

Jackie's Story

My son had hypospadius. We searched on the internet and realized the importance of being treated in a specialist team where they do lots of these operations and can prove they do them well. We didn't want someone who just does a few a year, and we were prepared to travel. I wouldn't bother shopping around for myself but you will go to hell and back for your children if it gets them the right care. A normal-looking, working penis is so important for a boy as well as a man. We talked it through with our GP and he found a specialist centre in London. We had exceptional care and Tom now has a fully functioning penis after a two-stage operation. Amazing.

Remember, no health service in the world can afford the highest standards of care for all its citizens, and in any one year by random chance alone, some NHS doctors, teams and hospital units will get better results than others. Half will always be below average, by random chance alone. But all should be above a basic, agreed, safe standard of care and should have their results closely monitored and quickly investigated if they fall below it. They also then need to be supported to improve the service above the 'safety' bar, or they should stop providing it if they can't.

In the English NHS, NICE is the organization that sets 'quality standards' for healthcare, social care and public health. They are well written, with versions for patients, and they tell you the quality of care you should be getting. They aren't (yet) legally enforceable – you are legally entitled to NICE-approved treatments but not to the highest standards of care by which they should be given. I think of the NICE standards as an upper bar of quality that you might get on a really good day in the right hospital unit or GP practice. But no-one has clearly defined the lower safety bar that all NHS services must clear. We do not have a National Institute of Good Enough (NIGE). In England, the Care Quality Commission tries to inspect everything (hospitals, GP practices, dentists, care homes) to make sure they're fit for purpose but the scale of the task is so huge, and their failures to spot poor care have been well documented. As a patient, you may or may not have the strength to decide what level of the bar you'll accept. If you or your carers are brave enough to speak up, the NHS must listen. Those on the receiving end of NHS care are the best smoke alarm it could wish for.

The three areas where British people are most likely to do their research, be assertive and seek out the right specialist care are when they are having trouble having children (fertility treatment), when their children are ill or need surgery or when they are seriously ill themselves when their children are young.

Wanting to be parents, or wanting to do your best for your children, are very strong motivating factors that overcome your traditional reserve and make you seek the best care possible. But as you get older, you generally accept what you're given or what's available closest to home. That may be because you simply don't have the strength, money or expertise to do the research and travel for treatment, it may be that you try and can't get a referral, or that you simply want to support your local NHS.

The best parts of the NHS are making it easier for patients to access and assess the evidence of what treatment is right for you, and who would be the right team to give it to you. Much of the 'performance' information is starting to be available online.

Imagine an NHS which automatically told you – without you having to go fishing – everything you needed to know about the safety and quality of the care, what the experiences and life improvements were of the patients who'd had that care, and how these compared with the average NHS benchmark. It would also link you to the website of the hospital, clinic, practice or community team where you could be introduced by name, photo and video to the people who would be treating you, they would explain what the possible treatments involved, the risks and benefits of different options and answer all your common questions. You could even join an online community of other patients and carers to exchange knowledge and tips about how to cope and get the right care for you. You could then choose and book your care at the click of a button, and be seen and treated within a guaranteed time.

This idea has been around for a while and if it was up and working, and patients were willing and able to use it, I wouldn't be writing this book. I'm a strong believer in transparency and accountability in the NHS, but it has to be done in a kind way or it backfires and makes the staff fearful and defensive.

I learned this the hard way. In 1992, I published the very poor results for babies having complex heart surgery at my local hospital in *Private Eye* magazine, because parents were not being told the truth and I believed it was their right to know that their children had a much better chance of survival, and survival without brain damage, if they went to other nearby specialist units. I was inspired by a very courageous whistle-blower, anaesthetist Steve Bolsin, who was telling as many doctors as would listen that too many babies were dying in his unit.

It was my decision to make this information public, and I naïvely thought this would lead to the immediate suspension of surgery, an investigation and a stop to avoidable deaths. In fact, surgery continued for another three years and it took Steve Bolsin going public and sacrificing his NHS career to get surgery halted. People at every level of the NHS, from hospital staff to the Royal College of Surgeons and the Department of Health had known Bristol had a serious problem, probably wouldn't have sent their own children for surgery there and yet sat on their hands while others unwittingly did.

Seven years after I published the very high death rates, a public inquiry was announced and I was summoned to give evidence. I thought I had simply done the right thing but as the enormity of what had happened unfolded, I started to have doubts. The information I'd made public was true, but I'd broken the story in a fairly aggressive, blaming way. This had the effect of making the surgical team and managers even more fearful, stressed and defensive ('We've got a mole!'), more bloody minded and blinkered, and determined to carry on. And the toothless regulators and Royal Colleges refused to stop them. So instead of halting the surgery and protecting babies, I may have contributed to more harm.

But by far the biggest shock for me was listening to the stories of parents. At the time I received several letters of thanks from parents who read *Private Eye* and had chosen to take their children elsewhere. One even wrote to the health secretary about her concerns, who bounced the letter back to the hospital. At the inquiry, it became clear that most parents hadn't the faintest idea what I'd written, and some felt profoundly guilty that this information had been made public, yet they'd missed it and their children had died or been brain damaged as a result. They felt they'd failed their children. Some marriages split up and two fathers committed suicide. I still feel a sense of guilt and responsibility.

When I gave evidence to the public inquiry in 2000, I argued that the NHS had to be completely transparent about the results of all its care, to collect, analyse and compare the data, and put the results in the public domain. It was essential to restore trust, for patients and carers to give proper informed consent and to travel wherever they wished in the NHS to get the care that was right for them or their child. Fifteen years later, heart surgeons at least have embraced this openness, are delivering stunningly better care and have action plans to intervene if a centre or surgeon gets a run of poor results. This information is available publicly, but isn't always easy to find. Most patients don't go looking for it, but are reassured that the information is out there and it's making surgical teams raise their game. The biggest gain has been NHS specialist centres sharing what they do, sharing results, benchmarking and working out how to improve their care, year on year.

One of the doctors leading the charge to openness is Ben Bridgewater, a cardiac surgeon at University Hospital of South Manchester (UHSM). Go to his page on the UHSM website and you can read not just his training and qualifications, but his surgical results and what patients think of him. There's advice on how to interpret the results and national averages for comparison. Some surgeons argue that results should be published for a unit, rather than an individual surgeon, as the latter might dissuade surgeons from taking on harder operations on sicker patients. An unlucky run of results could lead to an unfair suspension of an individual surgeon, and career ruin, so the temptation may be to become 'risk averse' and refuse to take on harder cases.

Other surgeons, such as Professor Ed Jesudason, argue that as well as publishing their results, surgeons should – with their patients' consent – upload videos of their operations to their hospital webpage and YouTube, and that patients should be routinely offered a video of their operation should they desire it. Jesudason believes that, as well as analysing results, patients can learn a lot about how competent a surgical team is by watching films of their operations.

In specialties where there are clear outcomes and fair comparative measures, such as heart surgery, doctors and NHS teams should follow Ben Bridgewater's lead and publish all the data patients need to know about experience and outcomes in a place they can easily find and digest before they have to make a life-altering decision. If you choose somewhere that does a lot of your procedure, does it well and the patients are happy, you can't go far wrong. For that extra cherry on the cake, look at the staff survey. If the staff in a hospital are happy working there, and happy for their friends and family to be treated there, it's one of the best green lights for great care you can find.

University Hospitals Birmingham has led the charge in allowing you to have your own personalized web portal with your records on it for you to access any time, share with others, get tips and tactics from patients like you, see the photos, names and qualifications of the staff who will be treating you and 'real-time' safety measures on your ward (such as infection rates, missed doses of drugs, falls and patient experience). Unfortunately, the hospital is now so popular it has currently had to limit referrals from outside its immediate area in some specialties.

Care is both what you experience at the time and whether your life gets better, worse or stays the same as a result of your care (the outcome). We used to either not measure outcomes at all, or just measure outcomes in terms of whether you got out of hospital alive, what complications of treatment you suffered or how active your disease was. Now we're slowly moving towards measuring whether your care or treatment allows you to do the things you hoped it would do in the longer term (e.g. climb the stairs, play with your grandchildren). There is evidence that those who have a good experience of care also see more improvements in the quality of their lives after care, but not always (e.g. you might have a wonderful experience of, say, a hernia repair, but it may have no later effect on your symptoms or quality of life afterwards).

If you're trying to track down great care, get as many sources of information as you can. What patients think of their care and treatment, whether their lives improve as a result, how this compares with other centres in the NHS and whether the staff would be happy for their friends and family to be treated there cover most of the bases. If this information isn't available online, ask for it. If a hospital can't or won't give it to you, you might want to find one that can.

Should You Pay to See the Right Specialist?

In theory, you should be able to go anywhere in the NHS to see a specialist whom you and your GP consider to be right for you, within an agreed waiting time. Problems can arise when your GP doesn't think you need a specialist referral, or wants you to see someone locally (possibly because of financial pressures from above), when you want to travel to a more specialist centre. There are huge differences in the referral rates and access to specialists in the area I work in (child and adolescent chronic fatigue syndrome) based partly on an individual GP's beliefs about the disease and whether he or she is allowed to refer outside the area if there is no specialist service locally (as there often isn't). We don't see private referrals.

Many doctors, medical trade unions, professional and health service regulators have private health insurance (sometimes as a job perk), so if those in the know are trying to buy themselves out of trouble, you may decide to do likewise. I don't have private health insurance but I would pay for one-off private care if I needed it and couldn't get access to the standard of care or specialist opinion I wanted on the NHS. I love the NHS and have been very happy when my family and I have used it, but I'm not prepared to die for it.

Some people try to use an initial private specialist appointment to jump the NHS queue and then slip back into the NHS for treatment. What you choose to do is down to your conscience, and the conscience of the consultant you see, but there is a company who claims it can – for a monthly payment – 'guarantee to get you in front of the best specialist within five days' without going via a GP. That puts a lot of responsibility on you to select the right specialist – or even to judge whether you need one – without your GP's expertise but if you can't agree with your GP, you might try it (although it sounds too good to be true to me). It's called as.one (www.betterasone.co.uk) and its strapline is 'better healthcare, guaranteed' – which seems a very bold statement from a legal point of view. And the promises get bolder . . .

> Our patients are diagnosed right first time privately, and then enter the NHS with a clear, informed treatment plan. One free private consultation is included in the membership each year. Our approach actually helps the NHS by reducing pressure on its resources. Less time-wasting visits to GPs. No inefficient referrals to the wrong specialist. No misdiagnosis and drawn out care costs.

There appear to be 1,200 NHS consultants endorsing this scheme in Scotland, England and Wales. Local to me, I know specialists in their own private chambers who are charging far less than the big private hospital chains to give patients quicker access to, say, MRI scans. And many NHS hospitals will now allow you to jump the queue if you can afford to pay to see a consultant or have treatment privately.

Like it or loathe it, the NHS in England is becoming more marketized, but buyer beware. In a financially incentivized systems there's a danger you will be given more tests and treatments than you need because each attracts a fee. So don't be fooled by the real coffee and the comfy seats. Keep your science head on and ask about the risks and benefits, expertise and outcomes before parting with your money. Doctors and managers are human and just as motivated by money, and the pressures of balancing the books, as you are.

Is It Better to Go Private in an NHS Hospital or a Private One?

The majority of private hospitals have no intensive care beds, some have no dedicated resuscitation teams, and surgeons and anaesthetists usually work in isolation – without assistant surgeons and anaesthetists in training present. There is often very little experienced cover at night, with typically one very junior doctor covering an entire hospital, and there are gaps in after-care too if things go wrong. On a safety-first basis, I would choose an NHS hospital if I thought the risks of complications were significant (there are always unforeseen risks too).

In September 2014, the Centre for Health and the Public Interest on patient safety risks in private hospitals calculated that 802 people died 'unexpectedly' in private hospitals in the previous four years and there were 921 serious injuries. It's hard to meaningfully compare this with safety in the NHS because private hospitals are still not required to make data on hospital deaths and safety incidents publicly available. Coding in private hospitals is often poor too but even without accurate data, the risks are obvious in an emergency.

The private hospital sector now gets over a quarter of its income from treating NHS-funded patients, so there is no excuse for not having comparable data available to patients about hospital performance and safety. The NHS still serves as a 'safety net' for the private sector. Thousands of people are regularly transferred to NHS hospitals following treatment in private hospitals, with over 2,600 emergency NHS admissions from the private sector in 2012–13.

Regulation of private healthcare in England is the responsibility of the Care Quality Commission (CQC), but the CQC can only make judgements on the data available (or lack of it). Records of clinical negligence claims against private providers are not publicly available, as they are in the NHS. And the Care Act somehow exempts private providers from the new criminal offence for providing false or misleading information to the regulators.

Patients using the private sector have no statutory rights to support complaints or to receive independent advice and support, nor recourse to the Health Service Ombudsman. And taking legal action for clinical negligence against a private provider is even tougher than in the NHS, where everything is overseen by the NHS Litigation Authority. A claimant against a private provider may have to try to prove whether it is the hospital or the individual surgeon or sub-contractor who is liable. For all these reasons, if you are thinking about going private, I would still choose an NHS hospital if it does not offend your ideology. It may well be cheaper too, although the rooms, food and views may not be as fancy.

If you're thinking of having treatment in a private hospital on the

NHS, ask about the safety net. What happens if there are complications in the middle of the night? Would they be quickly spotted? Would you be quickly transferred to the NHS if needed? Then you have to make up your own mind.

The Right Hip Replacement for You

- Newer is not always better.

- Choose a tried-and-tested hip.

- Choose specialists who can show you their results for the hip you've chosen.

- If in doubt, get a second opinion – it could be very different from the first one.

Hip replacements, when they go well, are one of the wonders of modern medicine. They can give you back your independence, free you from pain and get you back out doing CLANGERS. There are hundreds of hip devices, and thousands of stem/head/cup combinations. How can you possibly choose?

If you're having a new hip put in, should you go for one with an established track record, or a brand-new one with slick marketing but no safety data in humans? The choice is bewildering. Which of the 107 cups would you put with which of the 139 stems? A big or small head? Metal on metal, metal on plastic, metal on ceramic or ceramic on ceramic? A total hip replacement or just a resurfacing? Unsurprisingly, most patients let their surgeon decide for them, but as we discovered on page 62, two hip surgeons a few miles apart give you very different opinions about what is best for you. Get it right and a hip replacement removes crippling pain and restores mobility for fifteen years or more. When it fails – as 8,641 did in 2011 – it can be a disaster, requiring extensive, expensive and unpleasant revision surgery that isn't always successful. But if you ask ten different surgeons, you might get ten different opinions. So who can you trust?

In 1997, following the failure of the Capital Hip, I advised patients to choose a hip surgeon who used a tried-and-tested prosthesis and had a long-term audit to show he or she was good at putting it in. I also campaigned for a compulsory National Joint Registry (NJR) that published comparative data for all surgeons and the joint replacements they used, so that patients could see the evidence, and surgeons and regulators could spot a failing hip quickly and avoid unnecessary harm. The registry was finally up and running in 2003, but only in 2012 has it identified hospitals with the highest joint replacement failure rates. And it didn't stop surgeons in the UK putting in 10,000 of a 'brand-new' brand of metal-on-metal hip, the ASR, which has now been found to have a very high failure rate, requiring extremely unpleasant revision surgery in many cases.

Some orthopaedic surgeons may be wined and dined by the companies making hip prostheses, and some may have a vested interest in suggesting which one you should choose rather than which one is right for you. My advice would be:

- Do your homework. Look on the NICE website or the National Joint Registry and only choose a '10A ranked prosthesis', which should last twenty to thirty years on the balance of probabilities.

- Don't choose anything that isn't '10A', no matter how enthusiastic the surgeon, because history shows that most new prostheses fall by the wayside, and don't make it. Go for something that has lasted already. Better than taking a chance on a new prosthesis that might not last for five years. Treat any slight modification to a tried-and-tested prosthesis with caution. History has shown it may well not be an improvement.

- As for the surgeon, ask your GP and anyone you know who's had the operation. Avoid surgeons in their first five years of consultancy, and possibly in their last five years too. The best bit is in the middle, for surgical performance. Any surgeon who doesn't have anything to hide will show you their personal results for the type of hip you're considering from the joint registry, and how they compare with the national average. If they won't show you, or don't submit their figures for scrutiny, then run a mile.

- In summary: The Exeter hip is a good bet for most people. Cemented metal or ceramic head on poly cup is appropriate for everybody, irrespective of age and gender, but check it has a 10A rating.

- For very unusual, high-demand patients (e.g. athletes), willing to trade desire to be extremely active with increased risk of certain complications, I asked an expert. He said: 'Ceramic-on-ceramic hips and also potentially consider for large, young active males with excellent bone stock and normal renal function, hip resurfacing . . . done by a surgeon with a large number of hip resurfacings who can show he or she is good at it.'

- Currently, there is a huge problem with the fall-out from tiny design modifications to conventional hips as well as metal-on-metal hips, a huge amount of misery for patients and vast sums of NHS money being burned in litigation. As ever, better to get the right hip for you, right first time. And whatever treatment you choose, choose someone or a team who does a lot and can prove they do them well.

THE RIGHT HOSPITAL CARE

When I asked an audience of former hospital patients to come up with a checklist of things they needed to remember before going into hospital, and while they were there, I presumed it would all be about staying safe and clean. Some of it was, but a lot was about staying comfortable, eating, drinking and sleeping well, keeping in touch and keeping the home fires burning.

- Get someone to look after the cats.

- Do a big shop so there's plenty in the freezer for family meals while I'm away.

- Check work is going to pay me while I'm off sick.

- A map of hospital car parking, nearby car parks, prices and roadworks/closure updates.

- Notepad and pens to write down questions and important bits of information.

- A good book.

- Earplugs and a sleep mask.

- DVD player, music and really good sound-reducing headphones.

- Download the app that plays white noise.

- Lots of socks.

- Lots of pants.

- Own pyjamas and dressing gown.

- A nightshirt with 'Have you washed your hands?' written on it.

- Toiletries, toothbrush, toothpaste, floss, handwipes and facewipes.

- A very large bottle of hand sanitiser.

- Something to clean the sinks and showers.

- Family photos.

- My phone.

- Bananas.

- Make sure I can use the digital recorder on my phone in case there is something vital I have to remember.

- My laptop/iPad.

- Indelible pen to make sure they mark the right (or left) side.

- A list of all my medicines and diagnoses.

- Supplies of all my medicines to see if I'm allowed to take them myself.

- Names of everyone treating me and who is responsible if I have a problem.

- A note of how to contact the person responsible if I have a problem.

- A rota for friends and relatives so they don't all come at the same time.

- An address book so I can remind people to come and visit me if nobody turns up.

- A spare pair of glasses.

- A very obvious case for my dentures only with my name on it.

- Healthy snacks.

- Copies of my important medical records and letters, and a list of things that interest me and I like to do so my care can be personalized.

- My own bed.

- A clip-on water bottle and drinking tube so I don't die of thirst.

- Nutritious snacks to make up for hospital food.

- A note of my blood type and allergies.

- Check the staffing levels on the ward and get someone to stay with me if they drop below one in eight.

- Check every drug that is given to me, and make sure it's correct and meant for me.

- Check that anyone who tries to do anything to me knows what they're doing and can prove to me that there competent.

- Know the Twitter accounts and contact number of the chief executive in case I need to tell him what's going on in his hospital.

- Print out the NICE standards for Patient Experience and ask for them!

- Some cash to bribe the nurses if my care is really poor.

There's so much you could write down and so much you could ask, if you had the time and strength, and people were available to listen. You're more likely to be taken seriously by the NHS if you find out the official standard of care you should be getting, print it out, carry it with you and use it as a checklist to see if the standards are or aren't being met. Either way, you can feed back about your care in person, to the people caring for you, to the hospital and to the wider world (e.g. on the Patient Opinion website). It may improve your care or the care of those who follow. And never be afraid to ask questions.

One important tactic for surviving the NHS is to take your life and job skills with you, the expertise of anyone in your friends and family circle, and the motivation and determination to pull through for your family (i.e. a purpose to recover as fast as you can). David Grant was a senior project manager and coped with a very aggressive brain tumour by project-managing it.

SURVIVING AND THRIVING WITH BRAIN CANCER

David's Story
August 2005

'I'm sitting in my office and have a headache. It's distracting rather than painful but I have a lengthy meeting later in the day and want to be on top form. I pop across to Boots and spend 16p on a packet of Paracetamol. I take two, which sorts me for the meeting.

'I've been feeling increasingly tired but I've been working hard and I'm just a few weeks away from three weeks' leave, that'll sort the tiredness – I think. Back home in London I find I need to sit up in bed two nights running to relieve a headache. Something that hitherto, I've never been troubled with.

'At the weekend, friends come round for a barbecue. I don't feel quite right and in the early hours of Sunday morning I'm vomiting. I put this down to a virus I've picked up from Lauren, our two-year-old daughter. I'm not well enough to go to work next day but something is telling me to get an appointment with my GP, rather than just sit it out. I see his nurse, "Try a dairy-free diet for twenty-four hours." If I'm not better in that time, come back and she will get me in to the doctor.

'A day later and I'm no better, worse in fact. I return to the surgery with Lisa, my wife. I have little recollection of this visit but understand I was incoherent with my arm twitching badly. Dr Patel swiftly gets me admitted to St Mary's, Sidcup. Lisa takes me over in her Mini Cooper but on the way, is unable to prevent me from ringing the office and barking out some incoherent instructions.

'A scan reveals a possible tumour. Having referred the results to King's College Hospital, Saturday morning sees me dispatched by ambulance with the blue lights and siren on, over to King's. I'm making a bit of a recovery and quite enjoy the speedy journey around the crowded South Circular . . .'

In August 2005, David Grant was diagnosed with a very aggressive, fast-growing brain tumour called a Grade 4 Glioblastoma Multiforme. On average, only six in a hundred people are alive five years after surgery and chemotherapy. David had 12 good years after his diagnosis, and died in 2018. Having been unlucky enough to get brain cancer in the first place, he may have had genes that improved his survival. He was very fit, determined, positive and extremely well informed about and involved in his treatment. David meticulously 'project-managed' his brain tumour treatment, making very detailed notes along the way so he did not forget vital information. He published this log as *Surviving and Thriving. My Encounter with Cancer*, at www.braintumoursupport.ed.uk. Here are his reflections on how to get the best NHS care for a very serious illness.

Surviving, Thriving and Getting Better NHS Care When You're Critically Ill

'I do believe that mental approach is vital and here I was strong. I remember being on a stretcher post op thinking to myself, sort this Dave, you are a senior project manager, this project is important, it's about you and your family. You need a reason to survive and an inspiration behind you. My lovely two-year-old daughter was the powerful reason and my inspiration was my late father, who as a POW stared out the Gestapo for four minutes with a pistol at his head. It was the Gestapo that backed down. If he could do that, his son could deal with a glorified headache.

'Turning to my tips, in the absence of a centralized patient file, taking notes is essential. There is a requirement in many of them for the patient to speak out. This against a background of the British reserve re complaining. A way to combat this is to turn the complaints process into a patient feedback process. All the best companies use customer feedback to improve; creating a "what can we do better?" patient environment could transform things.

'There are a couple of things we all have to understand. The NHS. It is one of the largest and most complex organizations in the world, less than a handful of entities have a larger head count. For all its many centres of excellence its sheer size and complexity makes administrative failures somewhere inevitable. Major treatment will involve the coordination of efforts across multiple departments across several locations (in my case, starting with my GP, operated at King's and treated principally at St Thomas', it still involved treatment/visits to eight NHS sites. Coordination of efforts across multiple sites carries a high risk of communications breakdown, so be aware of this challenge and point out when it happens.

'Second point is understanding the underlying objective and reason why you are attending hospital. It is not to surgically remove a tumour, or to have a course of treatment, scans, blood tests, etc. The objective and purpose of the efforts of multiple departments is to restore the patient to the standard of health they enjoyed before medical intervention was necessary. Removal of a tumour is a surgical success but only a part of the restorative process.'

David Grant's Tips

1. **Keep good notes.** This can be a complicated process and there is not a file that follows you around so keep your own notes. Scribble down notes during the meeting, spend a few minutes writing them up when you come out of the meeting and type them up when you get home, while everything is still fresh. As your file builds up it will be more and more useful. It will give you real authority when you find

yourself being told something that just doesn't sound correct and you are able to flick back through your notes and say, "No, on the 14th Dr So n' So told me . . ."

2. **Stay close to your GP.** Your GP knows your medical history and you will need him to sign your off work certificate, so set up a regular meeting with him. You can use this meeting as a sounding board. I had a regular six-week meeting with my GP, or whenever I wanted.

3. **Arrive in good time for your appointments.** Some departments ask you to turn up fifteen minutes before the appointment times so that formalities can be completed, e.g. MRI scanning unit. Aim to arrive early for appointments. Trains do get cancelled and the patient before you could be stuck behind a broken-down train just as in real life. Being able to maintain a steady work flow helps everybody. The eye clinic St Thomas' had a sign saying 'Patients will not be seen before their appointment time'. Bad news for those that arrive by bus only to find they are stuck behind patients that are pacing up and down a South London train platform.

4. **Ensure your consultant is kept informed.** There is no central file following you around so when you have tests/treatments at other departments or hospitals check they know where feedback is to go to and by when.

5. **If you have concerns, raise them.** Speak to your consultant or nurse if you are concerned about anything. If you think it's something wider, use the hospital complaints procedure; you will find cards to fill in all over the hospital. Don't feel you are moaning, think of it as Customer Feedback. All the best organizations have it and deem it essential for improving their product/service.

6. **Can I help?** A consistent failure point was getting drugs from the pharmacy to the ward. At King's I was kept in an extra day to ensure that the medication I was to take home was ready. At St Thomas' promises of arrival in an hour, wait or pick them up tomorrow were never fulfilled. The solution, 'I'll go down and chase them. This is

always happening,' a nurse would say, 'No! Give me the prescription I'll hand it in and wait,' I'd reply. Contingency process worked fine and avoided taking a nurse away from a ward for twenty minutes plus. Don't expect everything to be handed to you on a plate, maybe there are some simple things you can do to help yourself and the NHS.

7. **Stand your ground.** You will build up a working relationship with your consultant but could have referrals to other units. If you encounter resistance, stand your ground. If there have been administrative failings, the one person not to blame is the patient. Ask for a matter to be referred to an individual's manager. Everyone you meet will have one. Report any failings back to whoever set up the appointment. When I turned up for my appointment for construction of the mask, the mask maker was keen to tell me how busy he was with many demands on his time. Additionally, it could not be done as the swelling was too great. I told him that my oncology nurse had guessed he'd say that and that adjustments could be made to the mask at final fitting. He relented and made the mask.

8. **Avoid getting involved in internal disputes.** Like any office there are factions wanting to criticize others. These are of no interest to you and are a waste of your energy. Ignore or report to your consultant or though the hospital complaints procedure. The NHS has high professional standards and you should expect to see them in everyone you meet.

9. **Take someone with you to important meetings.** There can be so much information that it can be difficult to absorb, another reason for taking notes. For important meetings, particularly early in your treatment, take a friend and debrief afterwards. If you missed or misinterpreted something, revert back and say so. Best to raise things early.

10. **Seek to determine points of outcome.** If you are being sent on a course of treatment, determine at the outset when the course will be considered as complete, by date or medical condition, and the points at which an escalation would be required. When my platelets crashed

to twenty-one during chemo, I was required to have daily blood tests (involving three hospitals) which could lead to a blood transfusion if they kept falling. They fell to fifteen before starting to rise. It was only when they started to rise again that I asked at what point I would have had a blood transfusion. The nurse needed to check but found it was if the count fell below seventeen, as it had the previous Tuesday. This error had no consequences for me but . . .

11. **Conclusion.** You are being dealt with by the largest and finest health service in the world. You should expect and receive the highest of professional standards. In instances when those standards fail, don't think of using the complaints procedure as a moan but as customer feedback that will get the NHS back to the high standards it expects to deliver. Besides, no-one has a monopoly on good ideas and you might just have hit on a good idea for improvement. Sometimes small improvements can improve things for everyone. If in doubt about anything, ask.

THE RIGHT BIRTH

Getting the birth experience you want, particularly when circumstances are beyond your control, is incredibly difficult, and not just for mothers, fathers and birthing partners but also for the staff. A wonderful midwife I spoke to sums up the current state of NHS midwifery services very well:

> The thing that frustrates me most being a midwife, is that we know what we could do to give families brilliant care and we desperately want to do it. But we just don't have the staffing levels. So the service has become a production line where we try to deliver a minimal safe standard of care where mother and baby survive unharmed, but we don't have time to put into building up meaningful relationships, getting breastfeeding off to a brilliant start, making sure the stitches are okay, etc. You know the parents want to ask you all sorts of questions and they want your time

and reassurance, but we have to send them home as quickly as possible. And some end up with episiotomies and C-sections that we may have prevented if we had the right staffing levels. Sometimes we have to close the unit and turn mothers away because we're full.

Birth should be a wonderful experience for everyone involved, but far too often you're just running around madly between rooms trying to keep all the plates spinning and hoping none of them fall. On the worst days, when there simply aren't enough bodies on the ground, I wouldn't want to have a baby on the unit I work on. I love being a midwife but not being able to deliver the standard of care I dreamed of when I was training is the biggest disappointment of this job. That, and the constant fear that we're going to harm a mother or baby by not spotting their distress in time. And that we'll be blamed and hung out to dry if things go wrong, and the 'system' will get off scot free.

Choice in childbirth is too often a joke. Too many low-risk mothers give birth in hospital when it would be safer for them to be at home or in a midwife-led unit, but they aren't supported. And that means the hospitals are overflowing and high-risk mothers don't always get the care they need, babies in distress aren't picked up, brain damage happens and 20 per cent of the budget gets spent on litigation. It's madness, but if you speak up you worry for your job.

Obstetric care in the NHS is as safe as it's ever been, and serious harm to mother or baby is rare. But harm does happen, and most of the NHS litigation spend goes on compensation for birth injuries. Even without harm, babies are put at risk every day by unsafe staffing levels – not enough midwives or experienced doctors on the frontline – and it's very common for women to say they were left alone for long periods during hospital labour.

New guidelines produced by NICE recommend that women with a low risk of complications in childbirth should be encouraged to either give birth at home or at a midwife-led unit. Whether the NHS has the staff to support this choice remains to be seen (the NHS is short of between 2,300 and 4,000 midwives to provide a safe service, depending on whose figures you believe).

The final decision about where to give birth is ultimately yours. You will never be forced to give birth at home or at a midwife unit if that is against your wishes, but you may well end up in hospital even if you wanted to give birth at home because there aren't the staffing levels to support larger numbers of home births, or because you or your baby show signs of distress at home.

The advantages of giving birth at home are:

- You will be in familiar surroundings where you may feel more relaxed and able to cope.

- You don't have to interrupt your labour to go into hospital.

- You will not need to leave your other children, if you have any.

- You will not have to be separated from your partner after the birth.

- You are more likely to be looked after by a midwife you have got to know during your pregnancy.

- You are less likely to have intervention such as forceps or ventouse than women giving birth in hospital.

However, there always needs to be a Plan B when you're having a baby. You may need to transfer to a hospital if there are complications. The Birthplace Study found that forty-five out of a hundred women having their first baby were transferred to hospital, compared with only twelve out of a hundred women having their second or subsequent baby.

For women having their second or subsequent baby, a planned home birth is as safe as having your baby in hospital or a midwife-led unit. However, for women having their first baby, home birth slightly increases the risk of a poor outcome for the baby (from five in a thousand for a hospital birth to nine in a thousand – almost one per cent – for a home birth). Poor outcomes include the death of the baby and problems that might affect the baby's quality of life. And epidurals are not available at home. Another risk of having a baby at home is that you feel so relaxed, you struggle to convince a midwife on the end of the phone that you are in the advanced stages of labour.

'HOSPITALS DON'T ALWAYS BELIEVE YOU IF YOU CALL UP AND TELL THEM CALMLY THAT YOU'RE IN LABOUR'

Gemma's Story

'How did you cope with the pain?' That's what people ask me when I tell them I had a home birth for Vicky, my first child. Actually, the pain was the easy part. The hard part was trying to persuade the two midwives allotted by the NHS to come to us to help my partner, Luke and I. It took seven and a half hours from our first call saying I was well into labour and three and a half hours from our call saying we were really in need of assistance from a midwife. They simply wouldn't believe me when I said I was in labour. But I was. I remember feeling afraid, telling myself they were going to come soon, surely they would.

If I meet anyone now thinking of a home birth, I say what I think. I think that hospitals don't always believe you if you call up and tell them calmly that you're in labour and need help. You need to scream, shout and go into a full *One Born Every Minute* act. Or your partner should. Otherwise, they may not come. Really.

I had a very easy pregnancy. I'd always hoped to have a waterbirth in a midwife unit. But during one of my earliest midwife visits, the midwife asked if I'd consider a home birth. I suppose, in that particular London hospital, I counted as low risk, as a lot of mothers there were older or larger or had various complications. I understand that hospitals try to recruit for home births as the statistics suggest that mothers who can give birth at home have less interventions – and the health service wishes to minimize Caesarian sections.

The idea did appeal to me. I read books and researched accounts, looked into countries such as Holland where home birth is the norm for all mothers. I decided to go for it – after all, if I couldn't cope with the pain, I could just go to the hospital – only ten minutes by car. It wouldn't take long for us to be in the maternity ward – and that epidural to be in my bloodstream.

Two midwives would come when I was three centimetres dilated – the same time when you are allowed to go into hospital. I'd have to deliver the baby in twelve hours or so otherwise we would go to hospital. The only thing that could go wrong, the hospital said, was if I rang up and there were not enough midwives to come out to me, so I would have to go into hospital after all. That would be fine, I thought.

Everyone thought I was ridiculous choosing to avoid pain relief. People clasped my hands and said, 'Don't you understand it will hurt?' I just said the truth – 'Look, I will try at home, and see how far I get.' I moved house across London and so had to move to another big teaching hospital, also ten minutes by car. They said they were keen to continue with the home birth plan.

A friendly midwife team of two ladies and a student came to the house, looked it over, left a bag of resuscitation equipment, told me to stop working and asked how I'd cope with the pain. I said I thought I'd be okay. I really did think I would. We hired a birthing pool, I read up on hypno birthing, did a short course on it and downloaded hypno birthing speeches. If I kept calm and told myself the pain was manageable, then I would manage it. I read up on theories of pain. I really did believe – still do – that the mind can have an effect on pain to a certain degree.

The young GP locum I saw for a check-up told me it was a dreadful idea and started talking about people giving birth on canal boats. I was a bit baffled. But I said to him that I would go into hospital the minute the midwives said there was any problem. I absolutely trusted them to see any such problem. They were the experts, after all. The baby was due on 7th August. By the third week of July, its head was so well engaged that at one appointment the midwife looked at me in panic and told me to stop working. But the successive weeks were pretty uneventful. I had no pretend contractions or any suggestions of final weeks' tiredness.

On 31st July, late at night, the waters broke, painlessly. Luke and I went to the hospital at 10.30pm, but I guess I didn't look much like a woman in early labour as the midwife on duty told me that if I hadn't started labour within a certain amount of hours (twelve?) I would have to have an induction. She said she'd book me in for an induction anyway. No examination was suggested.

We went home and to sleep. I woke at 1.30am and I knew there was no point lying in bed. The pain of the contractions was too intense. I went downstairs, Luke started filling the water pool and I listened to hypno birthing, did the breathing and did yoga poses. I threw up a few times and it seemed pretty clear that baby was on her way. Although the contractions were intense, they were manageable with the hypno birthing techniques.

I called the hospital at 2.30am and told the midwife on duty that I was in labour and so I might need help. I then joked that there was no need to have an induction and laughed a little. I am afraid I'm one of those people who often make little jokes in a crisis. It was a feeble joke – and I really see that joke as my downfall. The lady said that I couldn't possibly be in labour if I was laughing. She said to call back when I was in proper pain.

I think that I simply spoke too calmly – as I could talk through the contractions.

The call was a bit of a shock to me. I was expecting they would send the two midwives to me but clearly they assessed me as only in the very early stages of labour – when you're supposed to take a gentle walk and feed the ducks. But the pain was terriby intense. Still, I thought, if it was so early on, I wouldn't even be allowed to go to hospital. I'd have to stick it out. I got in the bath and started hypno birthing breathing.

By 6am, I was beginning to think that I couldn't cope any more. No-one had called us. Luke called the hospital. A midwife, Caroline, called me back. I told her that I was in labour, calmly. She said I was still in the early stages and should have a paracetamol. Luke called Caroline back on her mobile and asked her to come. She said she couldn't come as it was too early. We would have to wait. No-one timed the contractions or asked us to. They judged it on the fact I was calm on the phone – and people think first babies take a long time.

Luke called the hospital. They said Caroline would come when she could. He tried her again and there was no answer. I was by this point concentrating every ounce of being on breathing. I told myself what an idiot I was to think I could have a child without drugs.

Clearly, I was only a little dilated and couldn't deal with this pain so I would never manage to deliver!

At 7am, the nature of the pressure moved downwards from the stomach to the back and became more intense. I panicked. Luke called the hospital and told them this. The midwife on duty said that was fine, just meant baby was on the way. It's a key sign of course that baby has left the womb and is in the birth canal. (The head of midwifery at the hospital later told me this was the moment when I should have called an ambulance. But if someone's telling you you are not yet three centimetres dilated, you believe them.)

Luke kept calling Caroline and the hospital – but the hospital said the midwife was looking after it now and would come. She didn't answer her phone. By this point, I could barely speak and Luke was reading 'rainbow relaxation' over and over. The only thing I could say was to ask when was the midwife coming. He promised me soon.

Finally, nearly four hours later, the doorbell rang. I've never felt so relieved. Luke set off downstairs to get her and I got out of the bath and dressed. I was walking down the stairs to shake her hand when the midwife met me. Two midwives were supposed to come to a labour call. One – not Caroline but a lady called Laura – had come because we were not in labour. She told me to lie on the bed, just next to the bathroom for an examination. Then Laura said, 'Ah. I can see its head.'

I was a bit shocked. I said, 'You mean I am dilated?' She said, 'No, you're about to deliver.' There was no time to put down any towels or sterile bedding on the bed – or for her to get her gloves. Laura told Luke to phone Caroline, tell her baby was coming.

Vicky was nearly out by that point so Laura told me to breathe, not push. Caroline arrived just in time for the delivery of the body (as I said, you can reach us in ten minutes by car). Vicky was born twelve minutes after the first midwife's arrival.

But there was a problem. Vicky didn't cry and she was very grey. Her Apgar score was only two. Laura put her on my chest and rubbed her with towels. But no luck. She needed resuscitation. But the resuscitation equipment was downstairs in the room by the pool where I'd planned to give birth and it was still in the bag. Luke ran to get it and Caroline set it up – but that lost us valuable minutes. Laura told Luke to call an ambulance. It arrived while they were still resuscitating her and took her off with Luke and Caroline to hospital. I had to stay at home with Laura to deliver the placenta.

When Luke arrived with Vicky a full crash team was waiting for her. I arrived at the hospital about half an hour later to find Vicky in a special room, the crash team gone. Our little girl was looking pale and quiet but she was breathing. I asked the doctor if he thought she had been deprived of oxygen and if it would affect her. He said he thought she looked fine now and all the signs suggested she was fine. But he could not be certain. They then took her up to intensive care and we sat with her.

A further problem was that Vicky had arrived in hospital in a state of hypothermia as no-one had thought to wrap her up for the journey. It was August so not cold out, but one towel was not enough. The paediatricians at the hospital were very unhappy and asked me a lot about what had happened at the birth. They thought that the ball had been dropped, to put it lightly, by maternity services. They said I should consider complaining. I did mean to – but I was so focused on her in those early days and after we got home, I just wanted to forget. Also, the paediatricians, nurses and intensive care wards were amazing. I was grateful to them and didn't want to complain about the hospital of which they were a part.

We moved down to special care, then the ordinary baby ward. People were very kind to us. After a week, we took her home. It took us both a long time to get the hang of feeding and she was a rather nervous baby who didn't sleep much – but so are many babies!

I think now that the problem was she was in the birth canal too long – a good four hours. In the end, we cost the NHS a lot of money with paediatric stays. And surely that wouldn't have happened if she'd have been pushed out when she was ready to come out – 8.30am or so.

I did ask to look at my notes on the day we were discharged. I was interested to note that Laura had said Luke and I had rung the hospital and Caroline and said I was slightly uncomfortable. That's not true. We rang up to say we were in labour and wanted the midwives to come. But because I was calm, they didn't believe me. Who would ring a hospital to say you were slightly uncomfortable? Not me. You ring for help.

People say – but didn't you want to push? I think I did, but the pain control was so effective that I didn't really feel it. And I genuinely believed their diagnosis that I was not three centimetres dilated – and I knew you shouldn't push at that stage!

After ten minutes of looking at my notes, the head of midwifery and head of maternity services arrived at my bed. I can't say I wasn't surprised to see them. They asked about the birth, I explained what happened, they said I should have called an ambulance, etc. They were super sympathetic, told me I was a 'natural' at giving birth, said no-one should have said, 'You're not in labour if you can laugh.' They were very nice. But they definitely suggested that I had been rather exceptional in delivering so quickly and relatively painlessly – and so things had gone wrong because I was rather out of the ordinary.

I don't think that's true. I am physically ordinary. It was just that hypno birthing worked for me. And things weren't really that quick – just over twelve hours from waters breaking. The problem was that I didn't scream on the phone. I know that now. People might say – if that were me, I would have kicked up a fuss, shouted until help came. You'd be right. I should have done. But I am a rather non-confrontational sort of person and don't like to imagine that those who shout the loudest get what they need.

I can't say, however, that the experience hasn't made us wary about another child. I had a surge of hormones after delivery so didn't quite understand what was going on. But Luke did and he said he was sure Vicky was dying. There's no way we would have a child at home again – but we are even afraid of birth in general, when we were not before.

Hypno birthing really works. The principle of keeping calm and breathing made labour very manageable for me. But that practice of keeping calm and not crying out does mean you do not get the help you need. If you're going to do relaxation techniques, ready yourself to break out of them to scream on the phone or instruct your partner that he has to phone up shouting, 'My wife is screaming and says she cannot cope.'

We were the fortunate ones. Vicky was deprived of oxygen at birth, undeniably, but she's now a typical spirited three-year-old. Like any child, she's better at some things (spelling) than others (forward rolls) but that's just the same as I was as a child. I can't express how lucky I feel that we have her – and she has suffered no side effects of her birth.

Home birth can be wonderful with the right support, but there is a significant risk in the current NHS staffing crisis that there may not be enough midwives on duty to cover it safely, or that – as in Gemma's case – you may struggle to convince a busy midwife over the phone that you are in labour. We need to think about and address these issues carefully before we encourage more and more women to give birth at home.

One factor that strongly increases your chances of a good birth experience is a supportive birthing partner/buddy/doula. Dads can sometimes feel a little excluded from the process, but can be a vital part of speaking up to make sure your birth remains safe, and no unacceptable risks are taken. It's still very hard to do, but not impossible if you can think, explain and act clearly and correctly under pressure (TEA CUP).

Birthing Partners Are Crucial

'I JUST GOT MY MOBILE PHONE OUT AND RECORDED WHAT WAS HAPPENING'

Graham's Story

I wouldn't say that I'm a worrier but I am quite thorough, I do like to check things out. When Sarah got pregnant for the first time, I was delighted but also concerned, thinking ahead. Our local maternity unit has a bad reputation, and one of our secretaries had a terrible experience. She was left alone in labour for hours on end, there just didn't seem to be anyone around, then they got a junior doctor who didn't seem to have the experience and he couldn't cope and her baby suffered brain damage. She was devastated and it haunted me. She'd had a very healthy, happy pregnancy, really blossomed, grew a healthy baby and then they don't have the staff or don't follow the protocols or whatever to deliver safely.

Sarah was very keen on a home birth, in the water. I wasn't sure about the risks of that either, but I thought anything to keep us out of hospital. Then I looked into the risks and I found that nearly half of women who start off having their first baby at home end up getting transferred to hospital and our nearest one was you know where. I didn't discuss this in detail with Sarah, and she didn't know about my work colleague. We agreed that she would be transferred to hospital if her or the baby's safety was at risk, but she was sure she wouldn't need it.

I looked into Caesarian sections and forceps and all the other types of delivery just in case. I knew pretty well what might happen in an emergency, I knew the unit might be understaffed, I knew if we had a baby at the weekend the risk would be higher. I knew nationally there is a shortage of thousands of midwives, I knew that units sometimes close and turn women away. Maybe I knew too much, but I like to be prepared. I wondered, what would we do if we have to be in hospital and we are just left alone and Sarah or the baby is getting into difficulties?

My colleague's husband is quite emotional and I think it got aggressive during their delivery. I think that's understandable, and he was right to be worried. Nobody was listening to them and the baby ended up brain-damaged. But I'm not sure whether getting angry helps because often it just puts people's backs up and they don't listen to you. But what else can you do when you're frightened and you think your baby's at risk and no-one is listening to you? I couldn't see what the answer was.

I didn't share any of these concerns with Sarah. We joined active birth yoga classes, heard some mixed stories of hospital births and one or two great stories of home births. I could see why she was sold on the idea. Sarah had a complete belief in her ability to give birth naturally, she listened to hypnotherapy CDs, we got a TENS machine, we bought a birth pool in a box, what could go wrong?

She started having contractions at about two on Tuesday morning, which was good because it wasn't the weekend. We timed the contractions, called the hospital and by six in the morning things seemed to be underway and they sent the midwife over. She was about six centimetres dilated and allowed to get into the birthing pool. She was in, she was out, she was in, she was out, she was in a lot of pain, but coping on gas and air. Her waters didn't break spontaneously so they decided to break them but there was a trace of meconium, and the midwife said we would need to go to hospital. I wanted to discuss this with Sarah, but she wasn't really in a position to disagree – the pain got a lot worse after the waters were broken – and in any case a blue light ambulance arrived very quickly.

When we got to the hospital it was probably close to 8pm – I don't really know where the day had gone – it was very busy and the evening shift was on. We had a lovely midwife and Sarah was allowed to push, so she must have been fully dilated; she tried lots of different positions but the baby just didn't come. There were some dips on the heart rate monitor, which I spotted and pointed out, and they decided to get her into the theatre. I asked if this was for a Caesarian section, which was my preferred choice, but they said they would try forceps first. Consent forms were just waved in front of us, there was no real time to discuss, but Sarah was at least given a spinal anaesthetic which gave her amazing pain relief.

However, the consultant was then called out to another delivery and we were left with a junior doctor who didn't look confident to do the forceps delivery. The doctor didn't look at me and didn't introduce himself. So I asked him what his name was and how many of these forceps deliveries he had done on his own. He said he'd been observed doing some but this was his first one on his own. I said that wasn't acceptable to me, and I wanted the consultant to come back and either do it or supervise. I'd read about forceps injuries and the importance of having someone experienced using them or at least in the room. He said that the consultant was not available and that it would have to be him.

I was getting quite agitated by now, and really scared, and I thought I might pass out but I didn't let on. I just got my mobile phone out and recorded who I was, the date, the time, the fact that we were in the operating theatre and I'd asked for the consultant to come and supervise the junior obstetrician doing the forceps delivery of our child, because he had not done one on his own before and I did not feel confident that he was competent to do so. And that he'd refused to get help. The midwife asked me to turn my phone off in theatre but I'd got it on flight mode and recorded what I needed to record. The doctor looked absolutely stunned and then asked if I was a lawyer. I just said please get the consultant now. I didn't want to say I worked in IT. He left the operating theatre, and came back shortly with the consultant.

She briefly acknowledged me, did the forceps delivery herself, very slickly. It needed an episiotomy, our son was over ten pounds but born pink and healthy and crying and placed directly on Sarah for a cuddle. His Apgars were very good – I made a note of them – and he was wrapped up and given to me.

Did I do the right thing? I don't know. The labour ward was incredibly busy and you worry that by being demanding you are depriving another baby of a consultant's attention. But a dad's instinct is very strong, I'd done my research and I didn't want someone to do their first unsupervised forceps delivery on our child. We have since had a second child, at home, in a pool. It went like a dream second time and I recorded that too.

As a journalist, I've investigated stories of births gone wrong, and as a junior obstetrician who only ever wanted to be a GP, I've felt at first hand the horror of feeling out of your depth and not competent to cope in an obstetric emergency. In my experience, the quality of care we could deliver, and my own mental health, depended strongly on which midwifery team was on duty. If it was the A team, we often delivered great care. If it was the B team, it was decidedly mixed.

I could fill this book with stories that would make you never go near a hospital birth again. To get things in perspective, for every 100,000 births in the UK, 400 babies and nine women die. However, this varies dramatically from place to place, and in London the death rate for mothers is double. Many of the deaths would have been avoidable with proper standards of care. Obstetric units simply lack the staffing and experience to cope with so many older mothers and those with complex medical conditions and obesity. Harm to mother and baby usually happens when mothers are left alone for long periods, or a junior member of staff is doing their best in very difficult circumstances, without proper supervision. Neither of these excuses is accepted as defence if a case goes to court.

On a brighter note, the infant mortality rate in 2012 (four deaths per thousand live births), is the lowest figure ever recorded in England and Wales. I could not find accurate figures for brain injury. The British Birth Trauma Association estimates 10,000 women a year develop post-traumatic stress after their birth experience, and that 200,000 may feel traumatized by the experience. Clearly we could do better, but these issues have been around for a very long time.

Couples prepare for their birth in different ways. I recently met an obstetrician who'd been asked by a father whether he could have any training in recognizing obstetric emergencies. The dad was apparently a trained first aider, and keen to be part of the team spotting if anything went wrong with the birth. The consultant said he did not know of any such training for parents, but recommended a book called the PROMPT course manual, developed in the NHS but used around the world to help members of the team at any level spot and manage obstetric emergencies.

A few months later, the father arrived in the delivery suite holding the book which was very prominently displayed. He referred to it during the birth and asked lots of questions. Apparently it had a profound effect on the team and his partner had a happy, trauma-free delivery. Who knows how much reading the book or having it on public display affected the attitude and performance of the staff on duty? I suspect it was significant, and £26.99 well spent. More importantly, if you know how to recognize an emergency wherever you are on the planet, and have official guidance in front of you, you can use your observations and courage to save a life. Perhaps even two lives.

THE RIGHT JOINED-UP CARE

Illness can happen to anyone at any time, and it can stay with you for life. It makes ordinary people become extraordinary, as they live through hardship, savour the here and now and learn to join up their care with their life. You're never quite able to join up all the dots as you go along – living with serious illness is far too complex and messy to do that – but you can learn a huge amount from people who've lived well with illness for many years and want to share their experiences and expertise.

Wendy Lee got in touch with me to complain about an answer I'd written to a reader's question in *Reveal* magazine. Or rather, she tweeted that the answer had grossly oversimplified the impact Crohn's disease – a severe inflammation of the gut wall and much else besides – can have on a life, and I clearly knew nothing about it. I've spent thirty years encouraging patients to speak up, so I can hardly complain when they do. I sheepishly explained that I only had a hundred words to answer each question, but she had hit on the uncomfortable truth that I've barely been a patient in my fifty or so years, so what do I really know and understand about how to deal with illness and whether it's even possible in that frightened, anxious state to speak up? So I asked her to write her story and to reflect on what patients with a chronic, life-long, life-changing disease can do for themselves to improve their NHS care and fit it in with their life. She didn't disappoint.

'YOU CAN'T JUST SIT BACK AND HOPE THE NHS WILL LOOK AFTER YOU; YOU HAVE TO STAY ON TOP OF IT'

Wendy Lee's Story

I've been fighting Crohn's disease for control of the body we both inhabit for as long as I can remember. I was finally diagnosed in the spring of 1983, when I was nineteen, after seeing seventeen different GPs in my desperate attempt to prove I wasn't a neurotic hypochondriac causing my own gut spasms, diarrhoea and blood loss. The relief of being told I had a 'real' disease cannot be overestimated. The fact that I was told I must have had it for fifteen years for it to be in the state it was, was air-punchingly satisfying. From then on, I have to say, my care from the NHS has been fantastic. Everything Nye Bevan could have hoped for. But I had to work to make that happen as well. You can't just sit back and hope the NHS will look after you; you have to stay on top of it.

I've had ten surgeries since then, including an ileostomy (bag) and the following proctectomy to make it permanent, and to relieve me of the possibility of ever excreting the way nature intended. Without the NHS, I'd be dead. I come from a middle-class family, and before the disease got too debilitating I worked in creative industries and was paid well, but the cost of all the medical care I have had, the drugs I've been prescribed, and the bags and accoutrements I now need on top of those medicines, would have had us broke by now. The NHS is the jewel in the crown of this country, and we have to respect it – and hope like hell we don't lose it.

As a young woman, my NHS carers were mostly men in their forties, and their treatment of me was avuncular and warm. I was in and out of hospital a lot in those first ten years, so I got to know all the doctors and nurses involved in my care. I was younger than all of them, and did my best to develop relationships with them. That's the best thing to do – make yourself a person; open up so that they know you, discuss their suggestions, your treatment options, find out why you're taking that medication, having that surgery. You and they both need to be as well informed as is possible about what's happening to you.

I was lucky then, I didn't come across anybody who wasn't good and decent. Most doctors and nurses are good and decent; they wouldn't do those jobs if they weren't. When I was twenty-four, I'd had a few surgeries in quick succession, and my surgeon had left a central line tube in my chest so that they could give me TPN (nourishment – food, essentially) after any further surgeries. Back then, they believed in resting the bowel for a couple of weeks after resecting it (cutting out the offending bit of gut, sewing up the two remaining ends).

It was summer, I'd just met a new man (now my husband) and I was going to Edinburgh to meet him at the Festival, where we were both performing. I didn't want rubber tubing hanging out of my chest, and at the last appointment before I headed for Scotland, I demanded they be taken out. My surgeon was furious, told me I was doing it against his medical advice, but I was determined. He told me if I had them out, given my history of operations, I'd be dead within two years. So convinced was he of this that when I left, he phoned my mother and told her the same thing. So determined was I to wear strappy tops, I took no notice and the nurse took the tubes out. As I left, he called me back in. He told me surgeons sometimes liked to be proved wrong, and we parted on relatively okay terms. Sometimes you have to do what feels right to you. I was lucky that I was right that time.

Four years later, I got pregnant. My surgeon told me that wasn't the best idea, and that I'd probably need to be in hospital resting and being artificially fed (not sure how, given the tube removal) for the last five or six months. He was wrong again, and my son was born healthy and only slightly prematurely. He's twenty-one now, perfectly healthy, and as capable as any other young man of getting so drunk he throws up in a public place. He is my greatest pride.

Shortly after that, my GI consultant retired, and his registrar moved to a hospital in a different part of the country. I've always been lucky enough to be seen at a teaching hospital where I've had easy access to some of the best doctors and nurses in the field of colo-rectal care. If that isn't the case for you, do your research and find out who the best practitioners are within reach of your home. Don't leave it to chance, it's so important that the people looking after you know your condition. In the world of chronic illness, we have the time to locate the right people – it's not like we're going to get better before we find a good doctor. But even if you've done your homework, lived with the disease for years, know how your body works with it, things can still go wrong. Which is what happened for me around that time.

I saw a GI consultant who wouldn't listen to me. He was patronizing, rude and – crucially for me – humourless and dull. Once, he slid a bottle of pills across his desk to me and told me I should take them. When I asked what they were, he said they would make me better. I responded that I doubted that, that if they really would make me better, I would probably have been prescribed them before now. I didn't take them. He never told me what they were. On other occasions, he lectured me on how ill I was, and that I should stop pretending to be healthy. All my other doctors praised how well I managed, considering the Crohn's; I didn't like this alternative attitude. I'd argue with him in his office, then leave and cry in my car for ten minutes before I could drive home.

It took me two years of this before I wrote a letter of complaint to my long-time surgeon, and was transferred to the GI consultant I have now, with whom I get on famously. Of course, now that I'm the same age as the consultants, as opposed to the nineteen-year-old who was younger than the SHOs, relationships are different. At the hospital, my relationship with my GI consultant is the most important, but a close second is my connection to his nurse. With colo-rectal disease, in the bigger hospitals, there is a specialist inflammatory bowel disease nurse. Only one usually, these days, alas, but she or he is worth their weight in gold. Any issues I have, I go to her first, and she has sorted out a hundred things for me over the last twelve years or so. I have laughed with her, cried with her, and got several excellent recipes from her. She does this for probably a thousand other people, too, and I am careful not to bother her unless I have to.

It's worth remembering again that medical care is a two-way street. You have to be nice, be friendly, be yourself. Listen to the doctors; they didn't study for all those years and come out knowing nothing. We have to respect our carers if we want them to respect us. Most importantly, listen to your body as well, get to know how your illness affects it. Any good medical practitioner will listen to you as well as advise.

Their expertise + your experience = the best results.

With this in mind, when I decided – after four years in bed and myriad complications – to have a bag, I trusted my GI consultant to find me the right surgeon, once he'd got over the shock of my agreeing to have the surgery. As any good doctor would, he'd allowed me to spend all that time stuck in bed, venturing out only for medical appointments, until I got to the point where I knew having an ileostomy was the best decision I could make. And when I got there, he made it all as easy as possible. I had meetings with him and the surgeon where we discussed endlessly what the options were, and how we would proceed.

This was new to me – I'd not had any surgery for twenty years, and back in the eighties, patients did what their surgeons told them. That's all changed, and mostly I think it's a good thing. I'm much happier now I have the bag; my life has changed for the better, and I'm now only in bed for shortish periods, when I have flare-ups of the Crohn's. People are still surprised by that, thinking that the surgery should have been a cure, but I was never under that illusion. I'm still sick, but I'm not on the toilet up to twenty-nine times a day. I have to rest a lot, and the flares, when they come, are painful and sometimes crippling. But I'm good at being in bed, good at resting, and joyful that I don't have to do it all the time any more.

When you're diagnosed with a chronic disease, it can be terrifying. When it happened to me, there was no internet, no patient groups that I knew of, and to top it all, nobody had heard of Crohn's. Thankfully, it's all different now. There are official websites for most diseases, and they're worth reading for the factual stuff, but the most useful thing to come out of the digital revolution is patient power. You can find a forum for most chronic illnesses online, and they're a very useful first port of call for when you're newly diagnosed and frightened. Do be aware though, that people tend not to post when they're well – they're more likely to be enjoying a period of being 'able' – so you will probably find a lot of horror stories. It's worth knowing the worst-case scenarios, but hang on to how you feel, stay aware of how your own illness is affecting you, and don't get scared. More helpful, once you have a grasp of what you're dealing with, are patient blogs. There are lots of them out there – some well written, many not, but most of them useful. Also, if you find someone you feel will 'get' you, you can always contact them. I have made a couple of really good friends online through my blog and the forums I used after my ileostomy, when the whole bag thing was new to me. And I've blogged my experiences with my bag – from the decision, through both surgeries, to living with it – which I am delighted to find has really helped others.

After my second surgery, I had a horrible, terrible nurse. He was only on the ward for one day, but I have never felt so demoralized, bullied and disgusting as he made me feel. Foolishly, I never reported him, but I did blog about it, and as a result got a lot of feedback from nurses who were horrified. My point is, in all the many times I've been in hospital over the years, having a really unpleasant nurse happened only once. So shocking and rare was it, that I was moved to write about it. The same with the one terrible doctor, as previously mentioned. Only one of each. In thirty years of being treated for Crohn's.

If this happens to you; if you're not happy with your treatment, and you're absolutely sure it's nothing you're doing that's creating the problem, don't put up with it. Tell the practitioner you're not happy with them first, and if things don't change, write to one of your practitioners who you do trust. To make an official complaint is time-consuming and difficult, and you've got enough to deal with. Only do it if you are really not being heard by anyone else you turn to.

One medical person I haven't mentioned – the most important one you'll have – is the GP. It is from your GP that all your medical care will stem. If you're lucky, she or he will advocate for you, see you when you're in trouble, prescribe the medications you need – often having to fight to get them for you – and be your touchstone in the sometimes daunting world of the NHS. At least, that's what mine is.

After seeing seventeen different GPs at the beginning of my Crohn's journey, before finally meeting one whose sister had Crohn's and who instantly recognized my symptoms, I have been very lucky. Since that first brilliant GP, I have moved to a different area and have had two more, both of whom have been fantastic. I live in fear of my current GP retiring. I live in fear of all my NHS support staff retiring. We're all getting to that age. But as long as they're here, still practising, still being brilliant, I feel safe, and that's the most important thing of all.

In conclusion, if you're unlucky enough to be a member of the chronically sick gang, things are a lot better than they used to be. Listen to your medical practitioners, listen to your body, go to your appointments (the NHS loses millions a year over unattended appointments), take your meds (another source of waste – millions of people don't finish their prescribed medications), and talk. Keep talking. And keep listening. That way, both the medics and the patients will get the best out of the NHS.

Learning From Wendy

One of the toughest lessons of getting a chronic disease is that you've got it for life. You have to learn to live well with your illness. Wendy's courage and attitude are extraordinary in the face of such hardship, and her insights are invaluable.

Wendy was diagnosed with Crohn's disease thirty-two years ago, but she probably developed it fifteen years prior to that and it wasn't picked up by seventeen different GPs. Making the correct diagnosis is complicated and difficult in ten minutes. No doctor will get it right first time, every time. As we've already noted, a repeating theme in rarer and more serious diseases is that the diagnosis is sometimes repeatedly wrong, as one doctor might be swayed by what a previous doctor has decided, and delays in making the correct diagnosis and starting effective treatment can have very serious consequences.

When you've had bad experiences in the NHS, you have to learn how to trust again because there is nowhere else to go. This new trust has to be built on transparency and kindness, with you having the opportunity to question anything you wish to question. Wendy's story shows how the culture of the NHS has evolved over several decades. The old culture of paternalism and sometimes the dismissal of the patient's voice and concerns, has usually been replaced with a far more equal, open and constructive relationship – but not always.

Wendy describes the NHS care after her diagnosis as largely excellent, but this is partly because she is fully involved in decisions about her care and speaks up at times to get her care back on track and to make sure she gets what she needs, rather than what her consultant or the NHS thinks she needs. You may choose to sacrifice a higher risk of, say, a disease recurring or being harder to treat if your quality of life will be better. It's your choice.

To do this, Wendy needed to get to know about her illness, but also get to know the people treating her and make sure they knew her. Healthcare is ultimately all about relationships and collaboration, and if you're being treated by someone you simply don't get on with, it's far better to find someone else if you can. In over thirty years of using the NHS, Wendy has only encountered one poorly communicating consultant and one unkind nurse. However, when this does happen it's important to speak up to stop it happening again to you and to other patients.

Wendy's story also highlights the importance of being treated in a specialist centre if you have a rare condition. Not only will you see doctors with lots of experience of managing your condition, but you'll be assigned to a specialist nurse. Whatever chronic disease you happen to have, a good specialist nurse by your side is the best support you can have and one of the best indicators of high-quality care. The other vital indicator of good care if you need to use the NHS a lot, is to have a close relationship with your GP. Again, this might mean trying a few before you find one who you click with.

Patients Are Joining Up Their Care, in Their Own Way

Jacinta's Story

My daughter had surgery which went well but the ward afterwards was really understaffed, so I just sat with her all the time, guarded over her and questioned everything. On at least two occasions, I stopped errors with her medicines. I don't blame anyone – they were all trying their best – but I knew it wasn't safe and I knew I had to protect my daughter. I thought I would be too shy to challenge the staff but a mother's instinct is very strong.

Vince's Story

Most people say you need the support of friends when you're ill, but when you're an alcoholic and all your friends are alcoholics, you have to leave them to get better. My best friend is bright yellow and has liver failure, and yet swears he doesn't have a problem with alcohol. I want to be with him but I can't be with him, because it'll kill me too. I've had quite good care from the NHS and excellent support from my charity, but what will save my life is moving away from my old friends and making some new ones who are trying to save their lives and their livers.

Paul Wilson's Story

I lived on the streets for two years, and when I needed the NHS I got the best surgery money could buy. But the aftercare was useless, all they did was put me in a black cab and discharge me right back to the streets with some crutches and a bag of painkillers. I was really lucky I didn't end up straight back in A&E.

The really sad thing is my experience is not uncommon. Homeless people are often seen by doctors and nurses as disruptive and they themselves mostly just want patching up and sending on. But to end the spiralling cycle of careless discharge, crisis and readmission, the professionals need to properly think through what their patients are going to do when they leave their care.

How involved do you want to be in your healthcare? An NHS survey of a million GP patients published in December 2013 reported that 64 per cent said they are 'as involved in healthcare as they want to be'. Yet only 3 per cent had a care plan, an important document that everyone with a chronic disease or at high risk of hospital admission should have, to tell them how to best manage their condition at home, when to step up treatment if it worsens and when to seek urgent help. Given that over a quarter of the population has at least one chronic disease (15.4 million people in England alone), that suggests patients are accepting a fairly low bar for their healthcare, and below the standard the NHS sets for itself.

If you don't know what standard of care you should be getting from the NHS, you don't know when you're not getting it. Even if you do know, it can be hard to speak up and 'raise the bar' on your care, and you may have to keep repeating yourself and try to inch the bar up to the proper standard, little by little.

Writing about illnesses is a great way of understanding them and coming to terms with them, particularly if you swap stories. Many patients are already doing this on blogs, chat rooms and websites all over the internet. Wendy Lee's famous and wonderful blog is called My Baglady Life. The web is having a huge democratizing effect on medicine, joining patients up and sharing information. Many people find blogging about their illnesses, and getting feedback and support from others, is part of their therapy. It's also subversive. The balance of power is slowly shifting towards patients, but it still takes skills, confidence and courage to use this knowledge when you're looking after yourself or someone at home, or wading through the NHS. Being included in your care may not happen automatically. Don't be frightened to say, 'I'd like to be included in all decisions about my care, please.' Just get into the habit of asking to be included. The more you do it, the easier and more normal it gets, and the more the staff get conditioned to telling you.

Being included as not just part of a team, but as central to that team and with as much participation in decisions as you want, is fundamental to getting the right care. But the chaos of the NHS does not always allow it. You can do your research, know what you want, know what you should be getting, ask for it and still find it a struggle. Getting the right NHS care shouldn't have to be this hard, but sometimes it is.

'MY NHS JOURNEY WAS LIKE TRYING TO GET TO CORNWALL BY TRAIN IN THE FLOODS'

Jill's Story

I never know whether to laugh or cry when I hear people talk about giving patients power and handing them control of their NHS care. It's usually said by politicians who I suspect have never been seriously ill or used the NHS on a bad day. I've got not one cancer, but two. Pinky and Perky. One is hormone sensitive and the other isn't. I have no issue with the diagnosis, my GP was absolutely on it and I knew what I was facing within two weeks of noticing a lump. But the treatment's been chaotic at times.

With two different cancers, both in the same part of the body (can you guess?), I might have expected to see two oncologists. I've seen at least eight. I can only name two, and that's partly because they don't always introduce themselves. There is no named specialist in overall charge of coordinating my care that I've been able to find, although my GP does brilliantly to try to piece it together.

I've done my research. I've read my rights and responsibilities in the NHS Constitution and I know that patients who are informed generally do better. I'm frightened of cancer but more scared of dying before my children grow up. That is also a very powerful motivation for keeping me alive. So I learned as much as I could about my cancers, I read up on it on the internet on sites that my doctor recommended, the charities were great and I even bought a medical textbook. My chemotherapy was planned in advance and my GP contacted the hospital and went to great lengths to describe exactly the drugs I would be taking, in what doses and for how long, and gave me lots of good information. So far so good. I was an informed, involved and active patient!

When I turned up for my chemotherapy, I was met by a nurse who wanted to give me a drug I'd never heard of. The drug that I learned all about and consented to take had been changed by someone for some reason without telling me and they expected me just to go along with it. When I said I wanted to see the consultant, whose name was unfamiliar to me, this request was met with some reluctance. They were obviously very busy and had lots of patients to get through but this was a fundamental matter of consent to me. I was an informed involved patient. You don't change my drugs without telling me.

This was just the start of a very long journey. And not a smooth one, more like trying to get to Cornwall by train in the floods. Lots of big waves and high water, lots of hanging around with no information. You learn to always carry a good book and some food and water and, if you've got 'chemo brain', some peaceful music.

When you've got two cancers and you think you might die before your time, that gives you enough anxiety to be going on with. Time becomes very precious and you want to save it up to spend with people you love. You absolutely don't want to use all your energy fighting a chaotic system to ensure you get the treatment you're entitled to. But sometimes that's just the way it is. I eventually consented to have a drug that I hadn't been able to research, and it made me bleed. I went back to the oncology unit and asked them to sort it out. They told me to go back to my GP. I said, 'You're the one who prescribed me this drug, you're responsible for any side effects it gives me, you sort it out.' They said there was no-one there to sort it out at that moment. I said I wasn't leaving until they sorted it out.

I'm gently assertive and in control in normal life, but in the NHS and when you're ill it's different. I never get aggressive or swear, but I felt very upset afterwards that I'd had to stand up for myself and yet I kept apologizing to the nurses for having done so. I was in tears just asking to see the consultant. The clinic was heaving and yet I knew I had a right to be involved as a patient and that means being involved when things go wrong. Anyone who is sick enough to use the NHS regularly might recognize this picture. You can get brilliant individual care but if you're seeing eight different consultants, sometimes on different hospital sites, it's easy to slip off the radar.

I've had notes go missing, I've had vital test results and scans go missing, I've turned up for chemo and my name is not on the list, I've had a hospital refusing to prescribe the drug my GP has already prescribed because they can only give a cheaper version that the GP tried and it didn't work and gave me horrible side effects. I have to come to hospital regularly – four hours out of my day each time – to be observed while I inject myself with a drug. I've trained myself to do the injection, I can do it safely and competently and yet I'm not allowed to do it at home. I have to be observed in hospital for reasons I don't understand.

The biggest problem is that the system isn't joined up so communication breaks down. Computers don't link up, information doesn't get passed along and people don't talk to each other. I realized that I had to make my own copy of my medical records. Every letter that is ever written about me by a consultant or my GP about my illness, I keep a copy of and carry it with me whenever I use the NHS.

I carry a list of all my drugs, who prescribed them, what they're for, what the side effects are likely to be and how long I'm supposed to be taking them for. I use my phone to record memos of every important piece of information I'm given from whoever of the eight consultants I'm seeing at the time, and I use software to transcribe them when I get home and keep it in an electronic diary that I always carry on my iPad. You have to record stuff immediately or you forget it. The stress of illness, the NHS, waiting around, the fatigue and nausea and 'chemo-brain' play havoc with your memory. But with my own notes, I've been able to get my care back on track and avoid errors and duplications. I've been offered the wrong drug three times, and had the evidence to prove it. One consultant even asked me to email him a copy of my notes! How ironic is that.

So now I would say I'm getting good care and of course I'm grateful for it. Heaven knows what it's all cost. I think we should be told – and how much could be saved if we got it all right the first time. I've invested a huge amount of time, energy and emotion into staying on top of my treatment and correcting it. That's time, energy and emotion I wish I was spending on my family. I accept illness happens to all of us but having to work so hard to get the right treatment definitely wasn't in the plan. It's as if being a patient has become my full-time job. When you're ill, you just want to be believed, cared for and treated right. When you're not, you use what strength you have left to sort it out.

It would be wonderful to be treated in a kind, calm and connected system that gets it right without you having to continually check up on it. But I'm sorry to say it doesn't. Nobody can or will join up your NHS care as you're shunted from place to place but you. And heaven knows what it's like for the people who spend the last few months of their life fighting for drugs that have been denied to them. Life isn't fair but the NHS should be. It isn't always. I'm sure the people with the biggest brains, the loudest voices, the most status and the sharpest elbows get the best care. I hate to think that in fighting for myself and standing up for better care, it's meant that other patients are getting less time and attention. But what else can you do? Patient power shouldn't make me feel so guilty (that's another wasted emotion).

The one thing I would say is that it gets easier to speak up as a patient the more you do it. It's still uncomfortable for me, but it's much more doable. I think of it now like learning to drive or ride a bike. It can be very scary at first but your brain grows around it and, consciously and unconsciously, it gets easier. A porter told me somewhere I can always get a parking space, there are a couple of nurses – one of whom is always on duty – who I've got to know well and who 'get' me and can spot when I'm ready to blow. The receptionist told me where to get coffee that doesn't taste like dishwater. So it might be easier because I've skilled up and learned a few tips, or it might be easier because I've built up better relationships. But my care could still be a lot better than it is if I was treated in one team in one joined-up system all working together for me, not against me. And don't get me started on NHS wigs. PS: Please don't print my full name. I'm still having treatment. And I work for the NHS!

Learning From Jill

Life can be very unkind and unfair. You can have two or more cancers at once, and they may have spread even if you spotted them as fast as anyone could. You can be very well informed about your disease and the treatment you should be getting, and yet still find it hard to get it in a sometimes chaotic system. This isn't easy, and there are times when you, the team treating you and the system will fail.

If you work in the NHS (as 1.5 million of us do), you might think you get the perk of great care. This may have happened in the past – people got bumped up the waiting list as 'favours for friends', but much less so now. You may still use inside knowledge to track down what you think is the 'best' person for your knee or your pelvic floor, but you have to wait like anyone else and your care when you get it will usually be no safer or better. Many doctors and nurses I've spoken to have said they were powerless to correct failures in the care of their loved ones in hospital, even if it was the hospital they worked in. Many doctors now have private health insurance for themselves and their families, as do politicians, civil servants, and those who work for all the health quangos, unions and regulators – which tells its own stories about the pressures in the NHS. Although a private hospital is not necessarily safer and the last place you might want to be in an emergency.

Whatever health service you use, sometimes you have to dig your heels in and be assertive, even if it's upsetting all round. If you don't have the information you need to make an informed decision, keep asking until you get it. But don't get aggressive if you can help it and if you do lose it, apologize.

The person who prescribed your drugs is the person ultimately responsible for helping you if you get side effects. It may well not be that person who sorts it out, but it's worth keeping a list of all your drugs, what they look like, what they are for, what side effects to look out for, who prescribed them and how long you should take them for. Have it with you wherever you are in the NHS.

If you read the side effects leaflets that come with your drugs, the list tends to be very long and frightening, to cover every legal base. It may be easier to ask the doctor prescribing you the drug what are the common and important side effects to look out for and what you should do if they happen. Whenever you have a new treatment, always have a safety net in your mind if it doesn't work or goes wrong. If you develop a new symptom after starting a new drug, it's likely to be the drug.

The NHS Constitution tells you the rights and responsibilities of people using the NHS, at least in England, and it's worth reading, but you'll be surprised how many staff haven't read it. That tells you a lot about the culture of the NHS. There's a big disconnect between the centre and the edges.

People often use metaphors to cope with serious and complicated problems. Nicknaming your cancer can take some of the fear away. So can swearing at it, or looking at it under a microscope and drawing a picture of it (ask if you can). Meditation and mindfulness can sometimes help you cope with the side effects of chemotherapy. Music can take the edge off a busy outpatients but make sure you can hear when your name is called. Poetry and prose can give you inspiration, escape, purpose and meaning. Taking a friend and advocate nearly always helps.

In the NHS, important decisions may sometimes be made about your care without sharing them with you. This isn't deliberate, but you've either been forgotten or the task of telling you hasn't been specifically allocated to anyone. Remember the mantra 'nothing about me without me'. You are entitled to know, even if you have to go fishing to get that information. Call a time out on your care, or 'stop the line' until you understand it and are happy to proceed. This is particularly important to do if you think a mistake is about to happen in your treatment (e.g. wrong patient, wrong drug, wrong dose, wrong route into your body – or delays in giving you the right drug). Most harm in healthcare is caused by drug errors or delays.

Assembling and organizing your own set of patient health records, and recording and transcribing important information that various members of staff give you takes a huge amount of effort and energy. You may simply not feel up to it, or you may prefer to spend it on your family instead. Being up to speed with your treatment and knowing what you should be getting is good protection against poor care and increases your chances of getting the right care. Doctors have trouble storing this information in their heads, and someone who is fighting cancer and the side effects of chemotherapy almost certainly can't. Recording important memos on your phone is probably the least knackering way of capturing and keeping nuggets of vital information. Hospitals should provide facilities for you to record the entire consultation, but most don't. However, they should not object if you do it yourself.

A good unit will give you excellent handouts with all the information you should need to know about your treatment, who's giving it to you, what quality and safety standards they keep and how they compare with other units in the NHS. If they haven't, ask for these. If the handouts are barely legible photocopies, be on your guard as the hospital may not communicate well, and may not take quality and safety seriously.

Ask how much of your treatment you can have near or at your home. It can make a huge difference to the quality of your life. And it's worth asking several members of the team, as you may get different answers. Very high-tech care such as chemotherapy and dialysis can be given at home now, but as ever there may be a bit of a wait. So get yourself on the waiting list early.

Ask if there is anything more you can do to help to oversee your treatment. It may be possible for you to get important test results by email or text, and information that might save you a trip to hospital.

Keep your GP close to you and keep your GP in the loop. Communications between hospitals and general practices, and vice versa, are not always perfect. If you have important information that your general practice needs to know to add to your records, don't imagine the hospital will have passed it on immediately. Ask your GP if there is a secure email address you can send it to where someone will update your records. If your GP can give you access to your own electronic records, you may be able to add this information yourself.

Confidence and courage tend to grow the more you do something.

NHS care can improve in time, even if it gets off to a rocky start, as you learn new skills and knowledge, and you develop relationships with different members of the team. When you feel up to it, learn the names of everyone in the team who is treating you, from the receptionist and tea lady upwards. Make sure they know your name too, and slip in a bit of information about yourself that identifies you as a person. Find out about and show interest in them too. Personalized care does not happen by accident, you need to get to know the person you are caring for or who is caring for you. It's that two-way street again.

THE RIGHT CARE AS YOU GET OLDER

Do I really need to take these tablets? What would happen if I didn't? I mean, really?

John, seventy-eight

I hate taking all these drugs. I swear they make me feel awful. One day I'll open my bloody dosette box and throw them across the floor. I don't want to live forever.

Lucy, eighty-seven

I'm on blood pressure pills, because I hate the thought of having a stroke. They bring my blood pressure down to normal, I don't have any side effects and I haven't had a stroke. I'm thinking about statins but my cholesterol isn't that high and the benefits are more marginal than the blood pressure pills, so I've passed on those for now.

Phil, fifty-two

I'm ninety seven but I feel like a woman of ninety-two. I'm sure it's because I don't take any drugs. Apart from ginger wine. And I've never eaten junk food.

Ethel, ninety-seven

Help me! Help me! Help me! Help me! Help me! Help me! Help me!

Overheard in too many hospitals and care homes

In the UK, the proportion of people who are very old is growing faster than any other age group. There are currently three million people over eighty, set to double by 2030, and more people over ninety year on year. The number of centenarians has risen 50 per cent since 2002. The good news is that the majority of people over eighty say they are satisfied or very satisfied with their health, but many are frail. This isn't a diagnosis, but a warning that they don't have much in reserve. If you're not so steady on your feet, it doesn't take much to trip or slip and a fall can trigger a catastrophic chain of events leading to hospitalization and sometimes a permanent loss of your confidence and independence. The combination of physical and mental frailty is particularly high risk. Currently, 750,000 people in the UK have dementia, and that number is expected to double in the next thirty years. And remember, the NHS has a predicted black hole in its finances of £30 billion over the next five years alone. As services are cut despite rising demand, people will have to wait longer for care, get briefer, lower-quality care or in some cases be refused care.

The combined impact of this increase in life expectancy and frailty – and the budget deficit – on the NHS, social care system and unpaid carers has been huge. The majority of patients using GP and other community services are over seventy-five. The average age of hospital patients is over eighty, and 10 per cent of those patients are over ninety. The average age of patients admitted with hip fracture is eighty-four, of whom one in three has dementia, one in three suffers delirium and one in three never returns to their former residence. Most patients over eighty-five go to hospital because of an emergency, and stay on average for about twelve days. Some are never quite the same when they get out, but if they're given intensive physiotherapy and rehabilitation in hospital, and the same to welcome them home, they can be much more independent.

The majority of people nursed at home and who get help with daily living activities, such as washing, dressing and eating, are seventy-five or older. Older patients account for more than half the caseload of district nurses, half a million people receive home care from social services and 84 per cent of them are over seventy-five. Around 2.5 million people over seventy-five also have some kind of informal care at home from close family members, neighbours and friends. A quarter of carers are themselves sixty-five or older. Many elderly patients suffer social isolation and loneliness, which can be as bad for your health as smoking fifteen cigarettes a day. Many carers themselves suffer poor mental and physical health.

What Can We Learn From This?

We all get seriously ill eventually and we are all – at some stage – likely to become carers. It's the toughest job there is, and it helps to be mentally and physically fit yourself. To be a carer of anything (your children, your partner, your parents, your friends, your pets, your NHS, your planet), first you have to take good care of yourself.

There are huge individual differences in the health of people as they get older, which depend more on their physical and mental fitness, levels of activity and community engagement than their precise age. The more you can 'put in the bank' now to stay physically and mentally well, the more you will be rewarded in later life. You can never do enough walking, and those that do it for life have much better lives when they get older.

Anything you can do to prevent your mum or dad needing to go into hospital is worth trying, but it has to be with his or her inclusion and consent if at all possible.

The reason you may struggle to get the NHS care you need is because the NHS is caring for so many elderly patients with complex needs.

Older patients are not a burden on society. They are extraordinary company and tell the best stories. We need to take time to listen and to understand where our own lives are heading.

We all need to think about how and where we would like to die, and how much medical intervention we would like towards the end of our lives (knowing we can change our minds when the time comes).

Elderly patients admitted to hospital are often very ill – heart attacks, strokes, kidney failure, delerium (confusion), sepsis, chest infections – and most of these diseases are treatable. The key decision is whether you want the high-tech, pull-out-all-the-stops treatment of hospital – which can be scary and not without side effects, a bit like going over

the rapids – or lower-tech care in your home with more familiar surroundings but a higher risk of death. That death, however, may well be
more gentle and dignified than in hospital.

Even if the NHS puts more money into community care, the nag-
ging question for patients, relatives and NHS staff is, 'Could we be
doing more in hospital?' A better question is, 'Should we be doing
more in hospital?' Hospitals often aren't as safe and kind for older
people as they should be, because they don't always have the staffing
levels or structure for patients with such complex needs – even though
people over eighty are the 'customers' keeping them in business.

The vast majority of NHS patients are now older people – saying
hospitals are 'the wrong places for older people' is as ridiculous as saying hospitals are the wrong places for patients. They're the right places
for anyone who's seriously ill and wants high-tech treatment. They're
the wrong places when you're very ill, want lower-tech treatment
at home and are prepared to accept the higher risk of a gentler death.
But a home death is more likely to succeed if it's been planned and
talked through well in advance. For more, see Chapter 5, The Right
Death for You.

Agree plans and goals with your elderly relative. Decide on the level
of intervention you want in an emergency. Avoid hospital if you can,
but it's the only place to be for life-threatening illness if you want it
treated. If so, plan early to get home as soon as it is safe.

Look out for upturned carpets, loose rugs, puddles, power cables,
furniture on wheels, light bulbs that need changing and all those other
little things that could lead to a catastrophic fall. The internet gives lots
of good advice on 'fall-proofing' a home. But you still have to do it.

We all need to do CLANGERS every day, however old we are. Each
day should have laughter, purpose and meaning. Sharing stories with
those who have been on this planet two or three times longer than we
have, and sat with you through the real Clangers, is a great way to
CLANG. Talking to those towards the end of their lives is particularly
rewarding and enlightening. Some people save up some of their best
stories until last.

We all need to eat well, even if we forget we need to. Home delivery
of easily prepared foods is one option, and the delivery person can

provide company, check the microwave is working, check for uneaten meals in the fridge or freezer, raise the alarm if needed, etc. Some companies (e.g. Wiltshire Farm Foods) do a whole range of foods, with different textures for those with swallowing difficulties. I worked with them once, have been round their factory, tasted the food and would happily stock my freezer with it. I haven't been paid to say that.

It's very hard to eat with a sore mouth or ill-fitting dentures. Get this checked out.

Teams are vital in the care of the elderly, with carers and patients first on the team sheet. Write down the names and jobs of everyone involved, when they come, what they do and how they can be contacted. Make sure they all know about your elderly relative's death choices. You might be brave enough to stick them on the wall too, perhaps as a collage.

Ask to have one person in overall charge of coordinating the care (the team manager, often a named GP, with a named back-up). Remember to share. Care workers, physiotherapists, occupational therapists, nurses, GPs, friends, neighbours, food deliverers and family will observe and know things that no-one else knows, as will your elderly relative. Collect those nuggets and join those dots. Introduce yourself to all NHS and social care staff, ask about progress and goals, and feed back relevant information you've picked up. You should be part of 'a multidisciplinary team' with huge expertise to tap into. You may find you end up having to do a lot of the 'joining up' yourself. The boundary between, say, health and social care is completely artificial in real life – care is care, whoever gives it – but the NHS and social care systems still work as lots of separate tribes who don't always communicate, and it's often you who must bring them up to speed and plug the gaps.

Doctors aren't the first ones who pick up medical problems. You will have a good idea when a parent isn't well – trust your instincts – and all the other members of the team (particularly the care workers) may pick up early warning signs that could prevent a hospital admission. Do a SCAN or simply a problem list, and keep updating it so your GP can see how symptoms or problems have evolved over time, which ones are 'active' and which ones are currently under control.

The top five problem areas to think about are nutrition, mobility, pain, continence and mood. If you can keep these five on track, you can live well with just about anything.

For each member of the team, make sure they've heard your side of the story as well as your parent's. It's important to get a complete and accurate picture. If someone witnessed a fit, a faint or a fall, that testimony is crucial.

Older people can have really complicated medical care, but sometimes we make it far too complicated. An alarming number of hospital admissions are down to drug errors, interactions or side effects. Keep an accurate, up-to-date list of all the medications – what they are, what they're for, who prescribed each one and for how long – but more importantly do a regular review.

Most of us, whatever our age, hate taking tablets. But we collect them as we get older, and an older patient can easily be taking a dozen, or even two dozen, a day. For each one ask, 'Is this really necessary?' 'What is likely to happen if we stopped it?' Involve your parent in the decision. Some drugs are hugely beneficial, some have marginal benefits, some do more harm than good.

The more drugs you take, the more likely they are to interact and cause side effects, and we really don't know what the effect is of taking lots of drugs at once because no trials have been done. Most people, when they have the benefits, risks and uncertainties explained, opt for fewer drugs and learning to live with the symptoms they've got, rather than living with the symptoms the drugs give them.

When I worked on a care of the elderly ward, the wisest consultants would stop every drug they possibly could for an elderly patient who was admitted as an emergency. The vast majority improved, some remarkably. I worry that a lot of 'confusion' or 'early signs of dementia' may in fact be down to drug interactions.

If new symptoms happen shortly after taking a new drug, it's very likely to be the drug. Ask.

There is a lot of art as well as science in caring for an older patient, and the black and white rules of clinical medicine do not always apply. You will often get different advice from different professionals and you have to figure out which might be right for your elderly relative. Discuss it with them.

Infection is only worth treating if it's there. Most of us have murky pee as we get older, but far too many older patients are given trimethoprim or some other antibiotic because it's easy to put symptoms down to a urine infection. Urine infections are far more common if a catheter is in, so always ask if it needs to be in and whether it could come out. People need to pee, and if your parent stops, he or she may well need a catheter but not forever.

Keep your relative as active as possible. Walk and talk whenever you can.

Pain can easily go unrecognized among older people. Is your parent agitated and distressed? If he or she has painkillers and they work, laxatives might be necessary too, and should always be taken at the same time as opioid analgesia (codeine, morphine). Constipation can be more painful and distressing than the original pain.

If your parent is hard of hearing, get a referral for tests and hearing aids. You can also get an electronic amplifier as an app for your smartphone which you can then connect to headphones and improve the signal.

Does your elderly relative have the capacity to make decisions for him- or herself? It often depends on the decision. They may have the capacity to choose what they want for lunch but not which – if any – of five blood pressure medications is right for them. Find out more about assessing capacity and its implications on the Dying Matters site.

Falls and Pressure Sores

FALLS can be a disaster and can lead to a life-limiting loss of independence. Your'e most at risk of falling if:

- you have poor balance

- you take more than four prescription drugs

- you have muscle weakness

If you're elderly and have none of the above, your chance of falling over is 12 per cent in a year. If you have all three, it's almost 100 per cent. If you've remained active throughout your life, you're more likely to have good balance, good muscle strength and be on fewer drugs. Being active is the most powerful drug there is. Do it outdoors, be at one with yourself and the land you belong to and you may also stumble across peace, freedom, completeness and wellbeing.

PRESSURE SORES are a disaster when you're immobile, can be very hard to treat and they take up 4 per cent of the entire NHS budget.

The best way to avoid them is:

- Changing position as frequently as you can, with or without help. Every 15–30 minutes is ideal.

- Eating a healthy diet with sufficient protein, vitamins and minerals

- Getting enough fluid intake – www.hydrateforhealth.co.uk can help.

- Using a mirror or a carer to check the skin on pressure areas such as your heels and lower back – and asking for help as soon as you notice damage

- Getting all the help you can to remain continent and avoid prolonged skin contact with urine and faeces

- Quitting smoking – it reduces oxygen in your blood, weakens your immune system and makes pressure sores more likely

As in all areas of NHS care, charities are often life-savers in the information and support they can give you, for example Age UK, Alzheimer's Society. Often they can direct you to local services and activities. Your GP practice should also hold information about support groups. Being a carer is the hardest job there is, and you need to survive too. Respite care and regular breaks are key.

Consider taking on a personal health and social care budget to take charge of the money and directly buy the services you need. This has been a life-changer for some; others believe it could threaten the viability of the NHS (*see* page 214).

Many of these points apply to staying well in hospital. You have to be part of the team caring for your parent, and your observations and concerns must be heard. If you have a personal budget and employ your own carers, they can accompany you/your parent to hospital to be your advocates (*see* page 238).

Good care workers are life-enhancers and life-savers. For all the technology the NHS has to offer, there is no more powerful therapy than intelligent kindness. Healthcare without the 'care' is pointless and rotten, and a great care worker reminds us of the little things that make up great NHS and social care.

Here's a blog from a wonderful care worker called Emma Clifford. We will (nearly) all be carers one day, and we can learn a lot from it.

Ten Things I Know About Being a Care Worker

1. 'Homes Under the Hammer' will ruin your day because it will ruin the day of the people in your care. Unless someone has specifically requested to watch daytime TV, do everything you can to prevent them from languishing in front of that loathsome dross. Not just because it is soul destroying, but because the lack of stimulation and companionship would evoke anxiety or anger in even the healthiest of minds. The emotional impact is inevitable. If you really can't spend time with your residents because you're running around trying to make sure that no-one is thirsty/soiled/bleeding from a head wound, then do everything you can to steal a moment to put something interesting on. It's not hard to think of something more visually stimulating than the middle classes trying to make a profit out of the economic downturn.

2. Rome wasn't built in a day. I pride myself in being able to build strong, trusting bonds with the people in my care, but this is rarely achieved overnight. Years ago, I used to care for a gentleman who would only let me wash him; no-one else could get near him, and neither could I to start with. Then he let me give him a bowl of water to wash his hands in. Then he let me wash and apply cream to his feet. We chatted the whole time and the dry skin that had irritated him began to heal. After about six weeks we finally tried a full body wash and settled on a routine that suited him. This took patience, time and effort.

3. Good care workers are not meek and mild. We are advocates. We have to be able to speak up.

4. It's worth spending twelve hours' wages every six months on good shoes because your knees and back will thank you later. You may also want to consider stockpiling bananas and porridge oats. Each shift is like a workout: prepare for it and look after yourself. And, for the love of your stomach lining, don't fall into the Red Bull Trap. It's not pretty.

5. Care workers are vital. We are the eyes and ears on the ground. We know how much Mrs Smith normally eats and sleeps, if she's been this confused before, if she's in more pain than usual. We know what doctors need to know in order to make a diagnosis. We can mean the difference between prevention and cure.

6. It's okay to take risks but nobody really wants to say it. The only rule is that you must provide person-centred care, but we haven't worked out how to do this yet. Sometimes, I think we're scared of allowing quality of life, especially when it comes to dementia. Something might go wrong. There might be unpredictable outcomes, which would be terrifying. As a sector, we have a lot of growing and maturing to do.

7. I am a comedian. I did not know that you could dance to ABBA whilst sober until I started working in dementia care. I turn every-thing into a joke even if what I really want to do is go to bed and cry (or smack government ministers in the mouth).

8. Put yourself in their shoes, and do it properly. This isn't about bemoan-ing how hard it must be to have dementia/be in constant pain. Imagine what it would be like if it happened to you. How would you react? What would you miss? What would you get angry about? What wouldn't you get angry about? What tiny, little thing could make life just that bit more bearable? Now, research the person in your care. Use your imagination to piece the jigsaw together. Don't be afraid of trial and error. Remember, Rome wasn't built in a day.

9. This job will drive you mad. It's not just the lack of time, resources and common sense that will send you loopy. Nor is it watching

nonagenarians call out for their mothers, or wincing in pain that you can't take away. It's the 'up' side as well. I take genuine joy from my work, and laugh my arse off on a daily basis.

10. It's not all making tea and wiping backsides but both these tasks – and the humility and humanity to carry them out – are integral to the role. I have a working knowledge of five acts of law, a basic grasp of dementia-related neuroscience and intimate empirical knowledge of the effects and side effects of anti-psychotics. But if someone tells me there's too much milk in their tea, I make them another one. I hate too much milk in my tea – how would I feel if it was me?

THE RIGHT TO A BUDGET

In social care, people have been able to hold budgets to buy their own care, and initially got better care as a result, although the budgets are being tightly squeezed in the current financial crisis. When the same people cross over to the NHS, they're called patients and haven't, until recently, been allowed a personal budget for their health. But the benefits of, say, employing your own carers is that they can advocate for you in both the NHS and social care system.

In the English NHS, the current 'big idea' is to give patients with long-standing diseases and disabilities their own budget to buy both health and social care. You can interview and employ your own staff, choosing the ones that suit you. Being trusted to decide what's best for you sounds seductively empowering, but you've got to want to take on that extra responsibility, and have the ability to make complex choices and use the money wisely. And there has to be enough money in the system to make it work. Patients who've tried it already are generally very positive.

There are advocates and experts to help you choose, but ultimately the choices are yours. Most people with long-term illnesses and disabilities are good at difficult choices, and have to make decisions about what to do with limited resources every day. Politicians hope that if enough patients buy the nursing, physiotherapy and social care they want, along with wheelchairs and other aids to help them be more independent and live well at home, it should reduce emergency hospital admissions. It would be easy to set up a proper scientific trial to prove if this was so – recruit a few thousand patients who are eligible for personal health budgets, split the group in half and randomly assign them to either get a budget or not. Then follow them all up to see if the people with their own budgets have fewer hospital admissions. Sadly this has not yet been done. Research and reform rarely go arm in arm in the NHS. Enthusiastic ideology nearly always trumps evidence.

The risks of giving you your own budget to buy health services partly depend on whether you are just concerned with your own care at any point in time, or the potential impact on the wider NHS. If the money is taken out of the overall NHS pot at a time when it is already struggling (one suggestion is that £5 billion will end up in personal budgets), other services could suffer. If you decide to buy the services of a private nurse or physiotherapist, then that could either free up the NHS community services for another patient or plunge them further into debt because they needed your business. And if you end up buying services that don't work for you, you might feel that you are to blame which probably won't aid your recovery. As with much of healthcare and life, you end up making complex decisions based on imperfect information and you may have to choose what feels right and join the dots later.

Personal health budgets would allow more private health providers into the NHS, and they may come after your business – which you might like or dislike. In the studies done so far, people generally enjoyed having their own budget, it improved their social care, their overall wellbeing and quality of life but made little difference to health outcomes in the short term. More longer studies are needed, but politicians rarely wait for the evidence to arrive. They argue it is simply the right thing to do to 'trust the people' to buy their health and social care from whoever they wish, NHS or private. In Scotland, Wales and Northern Ireland they are far more wary of an open market in the NHS. Only time, and proper research, will tell us who is right.

To make patient-held budgets a political success, it's possible that the first people who jump at the chance will get a more generous budget than those who join the system later. If the money dries up when lots of people join, you may find it's a big hassle having your own health budget and you use it up too quickly. Or you may hand it over to a private company to manage for you. No-one can say how this will end, and we need more evidence to guide us. The scheme could give you more control over your healthcare and help you join it up – but at a cost. The patients who get the best NHS care may not be the sickest, but the ones who are best at managing their budgets.

NHS reform should be driven by evidence rather than party politics, but until we gather it your health choices may well be guided by your politics. Some patients refuse to go to a private hospital to have NHS care because they believe it deprives their local NHS of precious money. Some patients have died on NHS waiting lists even when they could have afforded to go private because they didn't want to jump any queue. Others absolutely love to go to a new private hospital on the NHS where you can park and get nice coffee and the staff seem so much less stressed. And many people with money – including doctors, NHS regulators and senior NHS managers – have private health insurance.

If you took your own health budget, you could decide only to buy back from the NHS, or you could shop around in the private market-place. Wherever you buy your care from, it has to be safe, effective, humane and right for you.

I'd like to see a proper scientific trial of whether personal budgets deliver value for money and improve lives before they are widely adopted. I'd also like to see a trial of 'navigators' or 'coordinators' of NHS care assigned to those with complex needs who want a first port of call to help them around a very splintered health and social care system. The right navigator could be the most important person in your NHS – you won't always be able to do it yourself, and neither will your carer.

THE RIGHT FEEDBACK

Steve's Story

My clearest memory of Sally's care was the way the doctor broke the news to her. He didn't introduce himself at all so we had no idea who he was or what his role was. He then kept pulling nervously on his

fringe and avoiding all eye contact when he told us Sally had a
space-occupying lesion in her brain. I used to work in customer
services for a large retail chain, and I just felt I had to give this doctor
some feedback. So I told him how important it was that we knew
who he was, what his position was and that he looked us in the eye
when he was giving us the news. We also wanted to know what
'space-occupying lesion' meant. He looked shocked, but by that time
I was used to dealing with doctors and not nearly so shy. When we
saw him again, later in the treatment, he came out to us both, shook
hands, looked us both in the eye and thanked us for giving him the
feedback. He said nobody had ever commented on his consulting
style before, so he thought he was doing okay. Sally's tumour was
benign, and she was awake when they removed it. I couldn't fault
their technical expertise – she made a full recovery – but I'd like to
think you can be a brilliant surgeon and a human being.

Constructive feedback is one of the most powerful and useful things
you can give back to the NHS, and other patients. If you keep it constructive and fair, it helps improve the service and directs others to
kind, competent care.

Another way to find the right specialist might be a 'TripAdvisor'
for the NHS. You need to be able to take a trip, so it automatically
disadvantages those who are too sick, or can't afford, to travel. But
transparency in the NHS – publishing outcomes – inevitably means
some people will shop around for the best outcomes.

However, honest constructive feedback, given face to face, in a drop
box or online, is an extremely useful way of helping to improve and
boost the morale within your local NHS. Ticking boxes is for politicians, your own words and stories are far more likely to lead to
improvements or reinforce and reward great care. And the more patients
who feed back, the truer picture we have of the NHS – wonders, warts
and all – to counter the overwhelmingly negative view coming from the
media. Here's one of my favourite patient stories of NHS care:

Everybody finds the GU (sexual health) clinic a bit scary. It just is.
For me it's a bit more than scary. I was sexually assaulted ten years

ago and find the examinations difficult after my experiences. After the assault I was examined by a male doctor . . . it was traumatic to say the least. Just to add insult to injury I have also had cells removed from my cervix (bear with me, I am trying to build up a scenario) so I have been examined by various doctors, nurses, blah blah. The point is this. Dr Bell is extraordinary. His approach, helpful manner and wit are second to none. I have NEVER ever felt so at 'ease' (relatively speaking) when having said examination. Having seen him twice now I can honestly say I will not see any other GU doctor unless I really have to. I was nervous the first time I went to his clinic; nervous about the examination and (wrongly so) the fact that he is, of course, a man! Pah! No female has ever treated me with such tenderness. I would like to thank Dr Bell and I meant to say it today but after my last visit I called my mum (confidant and aide) and cried (for quite some time) about the fact it was okay, that a man had dealt with me and it had gone well. I cried that my fear was over; believe me the police examination was horrific. I can't recommend Dr Bell highly enough. I never ever thought I'd get the chance to conquer the fear of a male examiner . . . but I did and he's the best :-) Who is in control? His patient :-)

A review of Dr Rob Bell on the iWantGreatCare website

I've worked in a sexual health clinic, and been a patient at one many years ago, and I have a lasting memory of how anxious, frightened, embarrassed and stigmatized you can feel. Removing that fear was the most rewarding aspect of the job. Dr Bell is, on this evidence, a very kind and competent doctor. He even manages some finely judged wit in a difficult consultation. But are you willing and able to travel to the Royal Cornwall Hospital to see him?

One route to great care without a huge amount of effort is simply to ask around. Tap into those learning circles. We do this in all walks of life to find a builder, a plumber or even a partner. I chose my GP, Dr Tim Sephton, after chatting to some friends in the pub. And he's brilliant. The school playground is another great seat of learning. The internet allows you to gather a lot more opinions of where to go for the right care very quickly. On the downside, you may well be putting your trust in strangers who don't know you as well as a friend, and they may have hidden agendas and vested interests. On the upside, if a lot of strangers say the care in a hospital is great, they're unlikely to be wrong. And the longer you stick around on a website or chat room, the more you learn to know people and trust their opinions (and learn who to avoid).

The NHS in England is becoming increasingly marketized, all hospitals and GP practices are having to collect and publish 'friends and family' feedback (would you recommend this service to yours?) and some hospitals even publish 'real-time' patient experiences from the wards to reassure you they're safely staffed and the care is kind.

If the information is honest, accurate, properly evaluated and published with the right motives, I'm all for it. The NHS has a history of data fiddling and there are all sorts of tricks to get patients to say nice things about you (e.g. ask them before they go home, when they're desperate to get out of hospital, rather than when they've had a few days to reflect at home about how good their care really was). I think the NHS should collect and publish its own patient ratings, but I think independent organizations or companies should do it too.

All feedback and rating sites rely on patients leaving honest feedback. In my experience, the overwhelming majority of patient and carers who leave feedback do it honestly, and it's extremely useful. The trouble is, not many of you do, so we may only be responding to the compliments and concerns of a biased sample.

That said, only about 1 per cent of customers rate hotels on TripAdvisor, but you rarely now see poo in a bidet or hairs around the plughole when you go to a hotel. The diligent feedbackers have raised the bar for everyone. However, if the numbers are small then it's easier for an owner to 'buy' a good rating or claim to be 'five star' on the basis of one review. Likewise, a vexatious complainant or competitor could sink a hotel with a few toxic reviews.

As someone who believes in transparency, I encourage my patients and carers to rate me in public. Putting this information in the public domain, on the iWantGreatCare site, provides important feedback to the NHS and individual staff, and guides patients about where to go to find kind, competent care if they want to go looking for it. However, be wary of the 'five-star' doctor or hospital on the basis of one or two reviews. Publishing patient experience information in real time, as many hospitals are starting to do, is a good smoke alarm to step in and stop poor care before too much harm is done, and a great way of praising excellent care.

NHS care is complex, and depends on teams and services as much as individuals. Patient Opinion is a not-for-profit service, founded in 2005 by a former GP called Paul Hodgkinson. It allows the patients and carers to have honest online conversations with NHS and social care services, whatever the standards of care have been. The best hospitals, GP practices and social care services respond quickly to criticism, investigate with meaning and share their findings. If you want to know what's happening in the NHS services around you, at least according to users of this site, you can sign up for alerts to be sent to you.

Here's an example of how it works when care is poor:

My mother is left needing the toilet for hours and ends up wetting herself and they don't wipe her clean or change her sheet. This is not a one off, it's a daily thing. Then she is left on a chair for hours because her bed is not made and no-one is in any rush to make the bed up.

Every day I have to take her clothes home to be washed due to the fact that they are wet with urine, from being left on the bed pan for hours. What a despicable thing. This is not a third world country. The staff I have met do not seem to be doing their jobs properly. It's so sad and upsetting. How people can be left in this state and people don't bat an eyelid?

Something needs to be done to make the right changes because this cannot and should not be allowed to go on. Shame on the NHS.

I'm so sorry to hear about your mother's experience and I would of course like the opportunity to investigate it further with details of where at the Royal Infirmary this is taking place. If you wouldn't mind contacting me directly, then I will personally ensure that the distressing concerns you raise are immediately resolved. Please feel free to get in touch so we can resolve your concerns. Please contact me on (phone number) or (e mail).

Kind regards,
Carole X, Director of Nursing

Remember too that all health services in all countries are facing similar challenges. Here's public feedback on the NHS website from a patient who used an English private hospital.

Things I Liked . . .

- The staff in outpatients were kind and understanding, as were one or two of the staff on the ward.

- The catering staff were very cheerful, kind and helpful.

- My surgeon was excellent.

Things I Disliked . . .

- Attitude of most of the staff was offhand.

- Drug safety (prescribed a drug to which I am allergic, drugs missed, staff not knowing how the morphine syringe worked).

- Poor cleanliness of facilities – and of me (as a patient who was unable to do much for myself).

- General neglect, including neglect of some essential instructions from my consultant.

- Found crying in bed by a visitor, where I had been for more than an hour, no-one on the staff had noticed as no-one had been in my room for hours despite me fainting the day before.

- Staff failed on a number of basic tasks, leading me to unnecessary discomfort and suffering which I could have done without.

- I needed some advice on aftercare at home (I had had abdominal surgery), but was given none at all despite asking two members of staff for it.

- When I rang up as I was bleeding at home, I got the brush-off twice on the phone before being called back to the hospital.

- Left hospital after five days in great distress with bedsores, a dressing which had to be removed and changed at home because it had been put on incorrectly, sore hands due to errors with a cannula, and a wound infection (wound still needed treatment a year later).

Anything Else . . .

- Under pressure from my insurer, I did make a formal complaint about my care a year ago. Since that time I have received (late) one sarcastic letter from the hospital, which I found very distressing, but despite me writing to them to say so, they have never replied.

If you searched for and found this comment online, it might make you search for other information before deciding whether to use that hospital. Or you might think that was a one-off, they were having a bad day.

The experiences and feedback of patients and carers is the best smoke alarm the NHS has for picking up problems and acting on them before they develop into serious harm. Increasingly, hospitals are using 'real-time' feedback, monitoring it and displaying it publicly. This is a great opportunity not just to flag up problems in your care but also to give positive feedback and encouragement. You need to blow the whistle on unsafe care, ring the bell for great care and help NHS staff improve the care they give you.

4

Trying to Put Wrong Care Right

When you look back after someone has been killed in a patient safety incident, you can often see that all the ingredients were in place for a disaster to happen. It was almost as if the person who died was a 'dead patient walking' as they stepped through the entrance of the hospital.
Sir Liam Donaldson, former NHS Chief Medical Officer

'I GET SO ANGRY WHEN I THINK THIS COULD SO EASILY HAVE BEEN PREVENTED'

Sally's Story

My dad has Parkinson's disease. He copes with it really well living on his own and manages all his medications. When he went into hospital, he asked if he could be in charge of his tablets and keep them by his bedside so he could take them on time. This is very important if you have Parkinson's disease as a missed dose can make you more likely to fall. The hospital said it wasn't their policy. They assured us he would get his medication on time, but the ward was so busy it simply didn't happen. He became unsteady on his feet, fell over and broke his hip. He never recovered well enough to go home and is now in a nursing home. I get so angry when I think this could so easily have been prevented if he had simply been allowed to be in charge of his own medication. He wasn't able to after his operation, so we set an alarm by his bed that went off loudly every time his tablets were due.

All humans make mistakes and NHS staff are no different, especially if they work in an unsafe system. We may also try to cover up mistakes if we think we're going to be blamed for them. In doing so, we stop others from learning from them so they don't happen again. My first serious medical error still haunts me. October 1986. I flushed an intravenous drip through with potassium instead of saline, having picked the wrong ampoule from the shelf. A rapid dose of potassium can easily kill by stopping the heart. In my defence, it was three o'clock in the morning, I hadn't slept for forty-eight hours and I was knackered. I had never put a drip in before and there was no-one to show me how. I was not brave enough to get a more senior doctor out of bed for something so simple. All I had was a book open on the relevant page. I wasn't even a qualified doctor, just a final-year medical student acting up to cover a junior doctor on holiday. I wasn't sure, and I'm still not sure, if that was legal. Identical bottles of saline and potassium were stored next to each other on the shelf, and the lighting was poor, I was sweating so my glasses were a bit misty and it was an easy mistake to make. But ultimately I should have read the ampoule properly. I was responsible for giving a potentially fatal injection.

This is how most mistakes are made in the NHS. It is usually one person who commits the final error, but there are a whole host of errors in the build-up, like falling dominoes, and a whole host of opportunities to stop the error in its tracks. We are getting better at double-checking, if the staff are available, but every patient and carer should check too when they can.

Fortunately, I was so incompetent back then that the drip had punctured my patient's vein. The potassium leaked into the tissue in her arm, rather than went to the heart. It was not fatal, but it was very painful and she let me know. I realized my error, paused for thought, and then told her she was probably allergic to saline. I hadn't even qualified, but I'd undergone the initiation rite of a doctor to make a serious error and then cover it up afterwards. One reason that doctors and nurses find it hard to raise concerns about others is that we've all harmed patients along the way, either by errors or substandard care.

I've investigated medical harm for twenty-five years, and I've found that people usually forgive honest errors if they are told about them truthfully. They may even forgive incompetence or substandard care if it happens once, isn't hidden, an apology is given and a lesson is learned. But people find it much harder to forgive cover-ups and lies. Deceit is profoundly unkind because it destroys trust, and the harm and anguish that follow are incalculable. This cover-up can continue for many years, and involve every level of the NHS from bottom to top. Vast sums of our money can be spent hiring lawyers to protect corporate and professional reputations, to silence whistle-blowers and to frustrate and cause huge anguish to patients and carers seeking the truth.

The biggest scandals in the UK have involved covering up poor care of the most vulnerable patients – severely ill babies, children at risk, vulnerable adults with learning disabilities and the frail elderly. These are precisely the patients the NHS was founded to care for and to protect with its ethos of care according to need. Patients with the greatest needs require highly trained staff to care for them, in sufficient numbers and working together without fear. Too often, they are let down and the staff also feel frightened to speak out.

These days, I've learned to admit to my errors. I apologize quickly to those who may have been harmed, and I discuss them with colleagues to work out ways of stopping them happening again. I also write about them and speak about them publicly, secure in the knowledge that I have an income outside the NHS – unlike most NHS staff – so I can blow the whistle on myself and others without losing my livelihood. I also share my errors anonymously with a centralized database. Such a database finally spotted that many patients have died over the years in the NHS because they've been given potassium injections by mistake. Potassium is now locked away in the drugs cupboard and the incidence of such deaths has declined.

No-one is quite sure how many patients are harmed or die avoidable deaths in the NHS. Research involving close analysis of medical records suggests in every modern health service, an average of one in ten patients suffers a medical error that might have been avoided with proper standards of care. For frail elderly patients the risk is nearer to one in three. Not all errors result in harm, not all errors could be prevented. One official estimate of avoidable deaths in the NHS is 12,500 each year but it's very hard to prove an exact number.

We don't know the true estimate of avoidable death because we don't put too much effort into measuring it and patients don't like to ask. But behind the numbers, each serious error is a terrible tragedy. I have twice been moved to tears at medical conferences. Most recently, it was hearing James Titcombe talk about the avoidable death of his baby son Joshua. James is a truly inspirational patient leader whose unstinting quest for the truth has exposed appalling denial, cover-up, self-protection and secrecy at every level of the NHS. James won't stop until the truth is told and the NHS has learned the lessons. Every relative I've met who has lost a loved one through substandard care feels the same. They aren't out for revenge but for understanding and constructive change to stop it happening to others.

Clare Bowen also moved me to tears with this speech at a conference on the need for openness and human factors training in the NHS, organized by Great Ormond Street Hospital. Her bravery, dignity and powerful message have stayed with me for six years, and will stay with me for life. It changed the way I practise medicine and how I think about patient safety in the NHS.

'WE WERE A NORMAL FAMILY OF FIVE; WE ARE NOW THREE'

The Bowen Family Story, Told By Clare

Good morning ladies and gentlemen.

My name is Clare Bowen, I am here today to talk to you about my daughter Beth, my family and how at 6.15pm on 27th July 2006 my family's world as it was ended. We were a normal family of five; we are now three.

I am not a medical person; the little that I know is learnt via three generations of my family being affected by the condition hereditary spherocytosis.

My father had his spleen removed over fifty years ago, my brother and I had our open splenectomies in the 1980s. Because of this family history and the knowledge you gain as parents of three children all affected, my husband Richard and I had gained a level of reassurance that the condition was manageable by an operation that is routine in any large children's hospital.

Over time new operative techniques develop and Will, our two-year-old middle child who had a severe form of the condition, was the first in our family to have the operation laproscopically.

The brilliant outcome of his operation and the improvement in his quality of life meant on our arrival at the hospital on 26th July 2006 with our five-year-old Beth, due in for the same operation, we had high expectations of an equally brilliant and successful outcome.

Beth, our eldest child, had a milder form of the condition, but was still tired and struggled to keep up with her peers.

Beth's operation was much more planned and we had met the surgeon who told us how the operation was going to proceed and how they were planning on getting Beth's relatively large spleen out through a Pfannensteil incision, so as to minimize visible scarring.

On the day of the operation, the junior doctor came to gain our official consent. 'Everything as planned,' he said, 'No need to talk about complications, they aren't going to happen!' We had an unusually high level of trust for this doctor (and the other surgeons) as they had all taken part in Will's operation.

We took our beautiful, amazing daughter down to theatre. We kissed her and said everything would be okay and that we would be here when she woke up.

But that was never to happen. Six hours after we had seen our daughter alive and happily talking away as usual, blood-stained surgeons, nurses and the anaesthetist walked into the tiny hospital waiting room, with no warning, to tell us:

'There has been a problem, something awful has happened.'

I had to ask the question, they could not say it.

'Is she dead?'

'Yes – we cut through a blood vessel and she bled to death.'

They were in shock. We were distraught, I was hysterical.

After a short time everyone left and at this point we were to all intents and purposes abandoned by the hospital.

Relatives helped us home; we then had to tell our three-year-old his sister would not be coming back. Richard said that this was the most difficult thing he had ever had to do.

Then bereavement services cancelled appointments that had been previously made by the nurses for us and no-one returned our telephone calls.

Four days after the operation we had had enough of being ignored and demanded to be seen, so as to begin to deal with the utter devastation that was around us.

My husband Richard and I arrived at the bereavement services office to be told there was nothing they could do as we lived outside the area. 'Goodbye and here are a few leaflets,' was their response.

We went up to the ward to collect a picture Beth had painted before she went to theatre only to find it had been thrown away. How could they not understand that everything Beth had ever touched had now become precious?

Then everyone appeared, doctors, surgeons and nurses.

We were sat down and told a very different story.

'The surgeon has just been at the autopsy and has informed the pathologist there wasn't enough blood for Beth to have died of blood loss.'

'The team have just met with the board we now all agree we don't know what happened.'

We left that day more confused, hurt and upset than ever. We went home to bury our daughter.

But as parents you can't leave it there, we had to know and understand why our daughter had died. At first there is a feeling of urgency that if you can understand you can then make it better and go back and fix things.

When your child dies your head knows they are dead, you have just organized their funeral but your heart does not yet know.

In your sleep you dream of ways to save them and in your waking hours you search for that question that once asked can unlock the path to bringing them back, as if you can dig up their body and make everything okay.

It took five months for me to realize Beth wasn't coming back. One day whilst driving I finally realized in my heart she was dead. This is why it is so important to listen sympathetically to parents and help them with questions; they are searching for that perfect question.

Eventually they will realize they can't bring their child back but even then they would give up all of their worldly possessions for just five minutes with their lost child.

The questioning later turns into a sense of protection towards your child, and as the only bit left is memories of them, you simply must know everything.

We fought for copies of Beth's notes which turned out to be woefully inadequate in places and revealed huge errors and incorrectly followed procedures.

We had a meeting with the surgeon and found out, little by little, more information.

They had been using a new piece of equipment. A morcellator. A rapidly rotating blade used to dissect organs internally.

The trainee surgeon was using it at the time of Beth's collapse.

It was the only piece of equipment in use at the time.

Beth's deterioration was rapid and complete.

We had to fight for every detail to be released. If we didn't ask we were not told. Richard and I were in way over our heads, neither of us had the level of medical knowledge needed and were given no-one to help us. It was very stressful and Richard could hardly sleep.

The hospital confused and clouded the issues and allowed us to follow irrelevant lines of enquiry so as to detract us from the main issues.

The hospital had thrown away the evidence that could give us a clear answer to what had happened: the bag in which the spleen had been, the disposable parts of the morcellator and most importantly the blood that Beth had lost during theatre.

They had not kept records that are compulsory in a theatre, such as the labels from blood transfusions given to Beth, so we had no accurate knowledge of how much blood she was given.

We were getting nowhere. The hospital didn't want to investigate. Our lines of questioning only led to more questions and the hospital was letting us fumble around in the dark.

We enlisted the help of a friend with medical knowledge to come with us to a meeting. Here things started to become clearer, the hospital finally had a qualified opponent.

We found out:

- They did not gain proper informed consent to use the morcellator.

- The operating surgeon had five minutes' training (undocumented) from a surgeon who had used/seen the morcellator in action five years previously.

- They had completed no risk assessment and had not followed correct procedure in implementing a new technique into surgery.

- They had made no attempt to retrieve the discarded theatre items even though they were still in the building and a surgeon openly said she realized at that point their importance.

- The surgeon with experience of this procedure was out of the operating area watching the view of the internal camera.

- This was only the third laparoscopic splenectomy the surgeon had carried out (Will's being her first).

- This procedure had never been done on a child anywhere in Europe.

Consider this analogy:

You are told your plane has a new piece of landing equipment on board and that a trainee pilot will use it. His co-pilot has little flying experience and had been trained on the new landing gear for five minutes by a pilot sitting in row five. Would you stay on the plane?

The difference between pilots and surgeons is that in a theatre surgeons do not put their own lives at risk. If, like pilots, they did then maybe they would be more keen to embrace human factors training, simulation training and briefing.

What mind-set did those doctors have that day to think they could carry out a procedure with no risk assessment or thought to human error?

Why did no-one in that theatre question the logic and safety of what they were about to do?

It was the surgeon's third ever procedure of this kind; did she not stop and think that maybe the introduction of a new technique was a step too far, that it would add extra pressure to the whole operation?

Before the morcellator was used the team had wasted forty-five minutes attempting to put a large spleen into a broken bag, they lost track of time and their environment at this point. On questioning, they estimated this part had taken no more than ten minutes and that if it had taken any longer they would not have continued to keep a child under anaesthetic for longer than required, and would of course have changed the bag.

But the video shows the correct time and proves doctors lose awareness and clarity of thought in such a situation.

The team had walked into theatre that morning, found the morcellator was free in the gynaecology theatre and a chance remark of 'How about using a morcellator?' resulted in a catastrophic tragedy.

The team had had a quick briefing, asked a nurse who had never heard of the equipment to put it together, and then didn't read the manual or safety instructions.

The manufacturer of this equipment refuses to put it into a hospital without giving formal training sessions to the users. They had it only because of its use in hysterectomy operations.

They decided to use a bag to hold the spleen whose instructions clearly said it was not to be used with a morcellator.

The team completed two other operations then turned, without further briefing, to Beth.

They didn't stop for one minute to consider our child.

Not one of them said, 'Hold on a minute, should we step back here and think about this?' If they had, maybe our daughter would still be alive today.

But the horror does not end there. We continued to hit brick walls and an unrelenting denial from the hospital with no open release of information. Being told once that 'information is not available to you, however if you have a legal team it would be'.

We finally appointed a solicitor, but the only way to afford this was to bring a negligence claim – something we never wanted to do.

I would just like to say at this point that I think I speak for the vast majority of parents in this situation when I say that the fight is never for a second about money. Why in the world would it be, what would you do with it? Build a new conservatory? Buy a TV?

We won our negligence claim, the hospital admitted they failed in their duty of care and we were awarded £10,000, apparently the value of a child's life. We paid for the installation of an adventure trail at Beth's school so that in a way she can still make other children happy.

A horrific three-day inquest followed. To sit there and have to listen to the events of Beth's surgery from numerous people was like being tortured with no possible escape.

Richard said he could not even leave as they showed pictures of Beth's autopsy. 'I failed Beth once, I won't do it again,' he said.

A so-called specialist was brought in. He had never seen a morcellator before, yet his evidence was held in the highest regard by the coroner.

He stood on the stand and said in response to the issue of consent, 'I use new pieces of equipment all the time, adding risk to patients, I do not see the need to inform parents.'

The coroner failed to get to the root of the problem, to uncover WHY this happened and human factors were never mentioned.

This is when I realized not all surgeons are the same. Some believe they do not make mistakes, therefore human factors training is irrelevant to them.

They are so detached from the patient that this has become arrogance and a misguided belief of infallibility that suppresses the needs of patients and their families.

I heard a trainee surgeon say under oath that he believed his five minutes of training on the equipment that day was sufficient. Who allows him to make that decision?

What is a surgeon thinking when he believes he can operate on a small child without thought to procedure and human error?

We all make mistakes. It is how we have prepared ourselves for them and then how we learn from them that matters.

Step back, think about what is happening. Involve everyone in the thought process: nurses, patients, families and the whole surgical team, and take things at a considered pace.

After the event all we wanted was the doctors to openly say, 'Sorry,' and not to be told, 'The hospital is sorry it failed to prevent Beth's death.'

And then for them to follow through with openness, compassion and honesty to the point of allowing themselves to be found at fault.

An event like this ruins the lives of families, the surgeons and nurses.

On February 12th 2008 Richard, completely out of the blue, died of a heart attack aged thirty-one, brought on by the stress of the preceding eighteen months.

I now raise two little boys on my own and will work tirelessly until all doctors understand human factors and incorporate them into their work every day.

We mustn't stop talking and discussing these issues until everyone understands that mistakes will always happen but we can minimize them and prepare for them with teamwork, training and support. And we must realize that telling the truth and treating everybody with respect after an event like this is all that matters.

Thank you.

A very moving film of Clare, Richard and Beth's story – to which I contributed – is available on an extraordinary website (www.patientstories. org.uk), which uses very powerful stories to provoke debate and generate change towards a safer, kinder NHS. Even though there was nothing Clare or Richard could have conceivably done in advance to prevent Beth's death, it makes us aware of how close to dangerous a lot of NHS care can be, and how we must all learn to be more careful and pause for thought before taking unnecessary risks.

I showed 'Beth's Story' to twenty-five second-year medical students from Bristol. They were all very moved (a few were in tears) and they all took it very seriously. Their thoughts were mature, insightful and in a few cases incredulous that this could happen. They were all glad they had seen the film, all felt they had learned from it and that it should be used more widely in medical training. They differed in their opinions of whether it should be made public, some fearing an anti-surgeon/ anti-NHS backlash. Many spoke of their admiration for Clare in her willingness to help us learn from Beth's story and to improve healthcare.

Clare herself took the film into the boardroom of the hospital where it happened. Her determination has made sure that Beth and Richard's deaths have meant something, and have changed the NHS for the better.

CAN YOU DO ANYTHING TO
STAY SAFE IN THE NHS?

Keep asking questions and keep speaking up if you spot something that doesn't seem right to you. The safest industries have a 'stop-the-line' policy where anyone can raise a concern and the whole team pauses for thought to consider it. Not all harm is avoidable, but everyone who works in and uses the NHS should be united in preventing the harm that is avoidable. Healthcare is fast moving, complex, dangerous and over-stretched. People sometimes lose focus, perspective and even the will to care. As a patient or carer you may sense when a ward or other NHS situation feels unsafe. In those circumstances, you need to be as vigilant and brave as you can.

If you're not sure what to ask in hospital (or anywhere in the NHS) read the SPEAK UP checklist, written by the Joint Commission in America (similar to the Care Quality Commission), an independent, not-for-profit organization that accredits more than 20,000 healthcare organizations. Its mission is for all people to experience the safest, highest-quality care and it recognizes the crucial importance of listening and acting on the concerns of patients and carers.

In a safe system, avoidable harm should never happen but, if you use the NHS, you'll know it simply isn't always safe no matter what the politicians tell you. The fact that it provides such good care to so many people is testimony to the wonderful staff, but even they would admit that the system is at breaking point and errors all too easily happen.

So what can you do about it? I hope by now you have the confidence to speak up in any situation, particularly if you don't understand anything and particularly if you think something is wrong. My experience is that patients and carers are often right, and I have seen many disasters prevented because they have questioned what was about to happen.

I have reproduced SPEAK UP below with permission, with slight amendments. The bottom line? If in doubt about anything, ask and keep asking.

SPEAK UP (or Ask, Ask, Ask)

Adapted slightly from the Joint Commission (www.jointcommission.org).

Speak up
Pay Attention
Educate Yourself
Ask
Know
Use
Participate

SPEAK UP . . . If you have questions or concerns. If you still don't understand, ask again. It's your body and you have a right to know.

- Your health is very important. Do not worry about being embarrassed if you don't understand something that your doctor, nurse or other healthcare professional tells you. If you don't understand because you speak another language, ask for someone who speaks your language. You have the right to get free help from someone who speaks your language.

- Don't be afraid to ask about safety. If you're having surgery, ask the doctor to mark the area that is to be operated on.

- Don't be afraid to tell the nurse or the doctor if you think you are about to get the wrong medicine.

- Don't be afraid to tell a healthcare professional if you think he or she has confused you with another patient.

PAY ATTENTION . . . To the care you get. Always make sure you're getting the right treatments and medicines by the right healthcare professionals. Don't assume anything.

- Tell your nurse or doctor if something doesn't seem right.

- Expect healthcare workers to introduce themselves. Look for their identification (ID) badges. A new mother should know the person whom she hands her baby to. If you don't know who the person is, ask for their ID.

- Notice whether your caregivers have washed their hands. Hand-washing is the most important way to prevent infections. Don't be afraid to remind a doctor or nurse to do this.

- Know what time of the day you normally get medicine. If you don't get it, tell your nurse or doctor.

- Make sure your nurse or doctor checks your ID. Make sure he or she checks your wristband and asks your name before he or she gives you your medicine or treatment.

EDUCATE YOURSELF . . . About your illness. Learn about the medical tests you get, and your treatment plan.

- Ask your doctor about the special training and experience that qualify him or her to treat your illness.

- Look for information about your condition. Good places to get that information are from your doctor, your library, respected websites and support groups.

- Write down important facts your doctor tells you. Ask your doctor if he or she has any written information you can keep.

- Read all medical forms and make sure you understand them before you sign anything. If you don't understand, ask your doctor or nurse to explain them.

- Make sure you know how to work any equipment that is being used in your care. If you use oxygen at home, do not smoke or let anyone smoke near you.

ASK . . . A trusted family member or friend to be your advocate (advisor or supporter).

- Your advocate can ask questions that you may not think about when you are stressed.

- Ask this person to stay with you, even overnight, when you are hospitalized. You will be able to rest better. Your advocate can help make sure you get the right medicines and treatments.

- Your advocate can also help to remember answers to questions you have asked. He or she can speak up for you when you cannot speak up for yourself.

- Make sure this person understands the kind of care you want. Make sure he or she knows what you want done about life support and other life-saving efforts if you are unconscious and not likely to get better.

- Go over the consents for treatment with your advocate before you sign them. Make sure you both understand exactly what you are about to agree to.

- Make sure your advocate understands the type of care you will need when you get home. Your advocate should know what to look for if your condition is getting worse. He or she should also know who to call for help.

KNOW . . . What medicines you take and why you take them. Medicine errors are the most common healthcare mistakes.

- Ask about why you should take the medication. Ask for written information about it, including its brand and generic names. Also ask about the side effects of all medicines.

- If you do not recognize a medicine, double-check that it is for you. Ask about medicines that you are to take by mouth before you swallow them. Read the contents of the bags of intravenous (IV) fluids. If you're not well enough to do this, ask your advocate to do it.

- If you are given an IV, ask the nurse how long it should take for the liquid to run out. Tell the nurse if it doesn't seem to be dripping right (too fast or too slow).

- Whenever you get a new medicine, tell your doctors and nurses about allergies you have, or negative reactions you have had to other medicines.

- If you are taking a lot of medicines, be sure to ask your doctor or pharmacist if it is safe to take those medicines together. Do the same thing with vitamins, herbs and over-the-counter drugs.

- Make sure you can read the handwriting on prescriptions written by your doctor. If you can't read it, the pharmacist may not be able to either. Ask somebody at the doctor's office to print the prescription, if necessary.

- Carry an up-to-date list of the medicines you are taking in your purse or wallet. Write down how much you take and when you take it. Go over the list with your doctor and other caregivers.

USE . . . A hospital, clinic, GP surgery or other type of healthcare organization that has been carefully checked out. For example, the Care Quality Commission visits hospitals to see if they are meeting quality standards. Ask to see the latest inspection report.

- Ask about the healthcare organization's experience in taking care of people with your type of illness. How often do they perform the procedure you need? What special care do they provide to help patients get well?

- If you have more than one hospital to choose from, ask your doctor which one has the best care for your condition.

- Before you leave the hospital or other facility, ask about follow-up care and make sure that you understand all of the instructions.

- Go to the Care Quality Commission (www.cqc.org.uk) and read more about the patient safety and quality standards at all the hospitals or clinics you could choose from.

PARTICIPATE . . . In all decisions about your treatment. You are the centre of the healthcare team.

- You and your doctor should agree on exactly what will be done during each step of your care.

- Know who will be taking care of you. Know how long the treatment will last. Know how you should feel.

- Understand that more tests or medications may not always be better for you. Ask your doctor how a new test or medication will help.

- Keep copies of your medical records from previous hospital stays and share them with your healthcare team. This will give them better information about your health history.

- Don't be afraid to ask for a second opinion. If you are unsure about the best treatment for your illness, talk with one or two additional doctors. The more information you have about all the kinds of treatment available to you, the better you will feel about the decisions made.

- Ask to speak with others who have had the same treatment or operation you may have to have. They may help you prepare for the days and weeks ahead. They may be able to tell you what to expect and what worked best for them.

- Talk to your doctor and your family about your wishes regarding resuscitation and other life-saving actions.

As well as speaking up, you may find yourself cleaning up dirty hospital bathrooms, taking in your own food, having your own drinking bottle close to hand – Hydrate for Health do a brilliant clip-on beaker and tube to stop a loved one dehydrating in a busy hospital.

CARERS ARE CRUCIAL FOR PATIENT SAFETY

Often it's left to the carers, rather than the patients, to speak up for patient safety, and here are some inspiring examples of those who've managed it.

Paula's Story

My mother has Alzheimer's. If you can deal with the behaviour without the medication and you have got experienced expert carers and nurses who are able to deal with it without the medication, obviously that's better. But there comes a point at which they do need medication and my mother is on medication and I think it is right.

I then think that the medication is not always monitored enough and I think as with my mother's case and I am sure with a lot of other people in a lot of homes the medication is used more than is necessary for the convenience of staff because it keeps people docile and it keeps them sleeping in their chairs.

And I realise my mother needed medication because she was distressed all the time and anxious and worried, so she needed something just to take that edge off. But when I saw her sleeping, sleeping, sleeping, and very confused, I thought, 'How much of this is Alzheimer's and how much is the medication?'

So I actually went to see her doctor. She is so lucky she has got this lovely young girl – I say young girl; she's probably in her thirties! – doctor, who is really nice and very thorough and very keen that we work together. And I hope I'm not a threat because we are nice to each other.

I actually made an appointment at the surgery and I went to say, 'I just want your advice but I'm not sure, I just wondered, I don't know about these things, but I'm wondering if my mother is very heavily sedated and whether there was any mileage, whether they could lift the sedation and, if that made her too agitated, whether there was some sort of anti-depressant because I know anti-depressants can work in a different way, they make you easier about life.'

She said, 'Oh I see what you're saying. I don't actually know but I'll phone the psychogeriatric specialist and have a chat.' The message came back that he thought it was worth a try and so that's what they've tried – they've lessened the tranquillizers, given her an anti-depressant as well and it may change tomorrow, you know, gradually it may change but at the moment my mother has got back a better quality of life.

So she's talking – she doesn't talk sense but she's got the energy to talk. She'll laugh, and when somebody comes up to her and says 'Hello,' she'll smile, and if they say something that's a bit risqué she'll go, 'Oh I don't know.' And that's how she used to be in the old days, so she's got back a little bit of herself by the right balance of medication.

So I think if it's possible you don't use medication at all. Obviously the professionals know better than I, when the medication should be brought in but I think there's a danger of it being used unwisely, indiscriminately if you like. And I think it's a shame that it can't be used more wisely and that there isn't, well I think it's like education isn't it – health and education are underfunded and under-resourced and undermanned. And in an ideal world if there were sufficient people to look after a limited number of patients then that sort of thing could be carried out. And I know in the hospice that's what happens.

I don't think my mother's medication would have been changed if I hadn't been there, actually. I think she'd have a worse quality of life. Yes, there comes a point at which medication is definitely needed because it would have been cruel to let her live a life of anxiety all the time and she was pacing and worrying and eaten up with anxiety so she needed something, it was just a question of the right thing. And people being encouraged to take the time and trouble to get it right. It seems right at the moment.

Angela's Story

My son, who's waiting for a heart transplant, had a portacath fitted three years ago due to his venous access being destroyed by a long medical history. I have had to train in how to access it because of the lack of nursing staff able to do so. I have had to argue with doctors about using veins instead, I've had to argue against a doctor trying to access the port with the wrong sort of needle (which would have damaged the port). One thing I hate is when my poor little boy is disturbed for invasive procedures whenever he's sleeping/eating/recovering from other trauma. I always tell the doctors to come back later and demand play distraction from play therapists.

Children would be abused in the name of medicine if it were not for 'bulldog' parents like me (and I'm fairly calm and neutral), but I've heard nurses complain about parents like that. I think the time the registrar attempted to access the portacath with the wrong needle was most clear in my mind. When I refused outright to allow either the port access or for them to attempt to insert a cannula in my (then two-year-old) son, he threw his arms in the air and stormed from the room. Eventually a qualified member of staff was summoned.

Graham's Story

My parents are eighty-three and seventy-seven, and for the past six years or so, my sister and I have accompanied them to all of their GP appointments. My dad has early-stage dementia and my mum has hearing difficulties. Both are proud people, and both have that innate faith that 'doctors know best'. Their combination of blind faith and minimizing medical conditions meant that they weren't getting the best treatment from a busy GP.

When my dad was still living at home (he's now in a good nursing home) and things were getting unsafe and upsetting, his GP said a marvellous, frank thing and it really helped me – 'You shouldn't have to provide all the care your Dad needs, but you are the facilitator of care.' That means, when I was getting rubbish support from social services and the NHS, he encouraged me to keep on challenging them. And sometimes you have to assertively ask for better treatment.

Mum now lives alone, and she has mild cognitive impairment. She is seen fairly regularly by a CPN, and she's prone to urine infections which affect her quickly and strongly (she gets very confused and can be delusional). This time last year, she was getting a bit run down, so we booked her into a care facility to get some respite (we hoped she'd get good food, company, exercise, etc). Within a week, she was showing signs of being delusional. The staff all assumed she had dementia. We asked that she be tested for a urine infection, but we weren't taken seriously. We said, she's had these symptoms before, she declines quickly – we weren't taken seriously. I called her GP, her CPN and social services. She was tested, and was diagnosed with a urine infection. But it didn't clear quickly, and she got worse. We were told to prepare for the likely conclusion that Mum couldn't live at home alone because of her mental state. We said, 'She has a urine infection, she's recovered before.' People were kind, but dismissive.

Mum then developed stomach pains while in respite care, a few days later. We were told mum was distressed and anxious. We asked what medical tests were being done. Again you get that look of, Well, she does have dementia and a lot of these people . . . We reiterated, She has mild cognitive impairment! We fought for her to be admitted to Ayr Hospital. After a week there, they finally diagnosed her with having gallstones. She hadn't been making up symptoms. She was given larger doses of antibiotics to cure the urine infection, and her gallstones were treated too. After a week in hospital, she was transferred to a respite hospital. She was still confused, but frankly, she'd been having a terrible time, with pretty shoddy care, so who could blame her for not being on top form.

The respite hospital advised us that Mum should move to a nursing home. I should add, Mum is adamant that she does not want to live in a nursing home. It's not her wishes. So my sister and I pledged to challenge everybody who said it's in Mum's best interest to move to a nursing home. She came home a week or so later. She recovered from that infection and gallstones, and she's still living at home – with carers popping in to support her daily.

The hospital staff were keen to see us as overly protective family members, refusing to see that Mum had dementia (despite the CPN team agreeing with us that she doesn't). They wanted a difficult patient sent to a nursing home. But we fought to get the best medical treatment for her. And we were proven correct. This time.

ACTING URGENTLY WHEN CARE IS
VERY UNSAFE OR UNKIND

In my experience working in and investigating the NHS for thirty years, truly shocking, unkind care is very rare – but it does happen. What is more shocking is that it often isn't picked up and stopped quickly, and it's left to incredibly brave patients and relatives to keep sounding the alarm until they're heard. Raising concerns in such a dysfunctional pocket of the NHS is very, very hard. Here are some things you could try:

Gather your evidence. Write down and stick to the facts. Missed drugs, dehydration, falls, soiling the bed and lying in it. Include dates and times. Support it with photos (e.g. of pressure sores, dirt, faeces). If you've already raised concerns about these issues and they have not been resolved, document who you told, what you told them, when and what happened. Include names and job positions.

Show your evidence to the most senior person available. Start with a clinician (doctor or nurse). In hospital, the name of a responsible clinician (doctor and/or nurse) should be above the bed of every inpatient, so that would be a good place to start. If the staff can't or won't put things right, and it's a weekday, take your evidence to the chief executive's office. Give the hospital one chance to put it right.

If your concerns are not acknowledged and addressed, and you still believe your loved one is in danger, take your evidence outside the hospital. Options include:

- Phone the CQC hotline (03000 61 61 61).

- Tweet your concerns, with or without a photo, copying the hospital and the chief executive if they have Twitter accounts.

- Use Patient Opinion or one of the other public feedback websites.

- Tell your MP, GP and clinical commissioning group.

- Tell the local and national media.

- Try other helplines: NHS Complaints Advocacy helpline 0300 330 5454, NHS England complaints helpline 0300 311 2233 and the Ombudsman complaints helpline 0345 015 4033. All are weekday working hours only.

These extreme measures are needed in extreme circumstances. At Stafford Hospitals run by Mid Staffordshire NHS Hospital Trust, great care coexisted alongside truly appalling care. An elderly man forced to stay on a commode for fifty-five minutes wearing only a pyjama top; a woman whose legs were 'red raw' because of the effect of her uncleaned faeces; piles of soiled sheets and vomit bowls left at the end of beds; a woman arrived at 10am to find her ninety-six-year-old mother-in-law 'completely naked . . . and covered with faeces . . . It was in her hair, her nails, her hands and on all the cot sides . . . it was literally everywhere and it was dried.' Another woman who found her mother with faeces under her nails asked for them to be cut, but was told that it was 'not in the nurses' remit to cut patients' nails'.

Such negligent 'care' is rare, but it does happen and each year the Patients Association (I'm a Vice President) highlights it. I asked the Care Quality Commission for their official advice – here's CQC's advice on what to do if someone is at risk of harm in a care setting:

If possible, raise your concern with provider staff and/or local and more senior managers, through face-to-face contact and then formal procedures as needed in the circumstances. Providers have internal procedures by which service users/patients, their families, friends and carers, the public and staff can raise concerns.

If your concern relates to a particularly urgent situation involving immediate avoidable harm and/or abuse, and for whatever reason it is not appropriate to approach staff at the provider for help (or you have done so but still feel someone is at serious risk), then contact the relevant emergency service(s).

If you are concerned about abuse or alleged abuse but it is not appropriate to call in the emergency services or contact the provider or its staff, raise your concerns with the relevant local authority safeguarding team, for adults or children as relevant.

If there are reasons why a person feels unable to take the actions above, they can contact CQC by telephone (03000 61 61 61), listen to the opening message, and select the appropriate service (option 2) to immediately be put through to our safety escalation team. They can also email us at Enquiries@cqc.org.uk, contact us via our online form or write to us at CQC National Customer Service Centre, Citygate, Gallowgate, Newcastle upon Tyne NE1 4PA. Please note, however, that our telephone opening hours are Monday to Friday between 8.30am and 5.30pm.

People should use the provider's internal procedures rather than call the emergency services if at all possible in urgent situations. Calling the emergency services is an extreme measure and should only be considered if this is in the best interests of the patient and would not cause further harm. However, if internal processes fail or cannot be used for some reason then they may wish to use the emergency services as a last resort.

Julie Bailey's mother Bella died at Stafford Hospital in appalling circumstances. She founded Cure the NHS, supported others with similar experiences and campaigned for a public inquiry. Despite all the official guidance, her story shows how hard it is to be listened to and taken seriously when a part of the NHS is in denial and nobody appears to be accountable for the poor care:

When I came out of the hospital I thought that I would just have to tell people and something would be done about it. Instead, a small group of mostly elderly people had to stand out in the wind, snow and rain for nearly two years following Ministers round to try and get the public inquiry.

Here is Julie's advice to those in a similar position:

- When something goes wrong a person is not in a position to be searching around for information and to find out who to approach. The secret is to tell as many people as possible as quickly as possible and not to be fobbed off; be persistent, as not doing enough may be something you regret forever. The press really are key and a call from an inquisitive journalist always does the trick, in my experience.

- I rarely advise anyone to call the police. I have found that they have never supported the patient/relative, but tend to side with the hospital. Perhaps the police would help more if there was legislation but at the moment the legal system is lacking. I was hoping that from the public inquiry we could come up with a set procedure for MPs, GPs, CCGs etc. to take up complaints to help patients/relatives but that hasn't happened. And they are still doing their own thing, some are helpful but others side with the hospital, particularly GPs.

- I'm finding that Twitter is a great way of getting chief executives to respond to complainants. I think there are huge problems with PALS and the complaints system, and once CEOs become aware of a problem they want to help.

- If a family rings me and their family member is on a ward, the priority usually is to do something quickly, to stop any further deterioration. I tend to find it is usually a weekend or evening and I advise them to ask to speak to the person responsible for the hospital, in the chief executive's absence. If the responsible person is not clinical, I advise them to ask for the medical or nursing director to be contacted. Using the press as a threat usually works and once a hospital knows that I am involved, they fear the national press. The NHS just hates bad publicity and I have found that it is really the only thing that has such an impact.

- I advise people to write everything down, get a witness, even if it's another patient, but to avoid relatives/friends if they can help it, someone independent is preferable. Evidence is critical and I advise people to take pictures of anything suspicious and that includes medical records. Take pictures of them regularly to keep a record just in case they are needed.

- I examined about a hundred case notes from Mid Staffs victims that had been tampered with and that seemed to happen as soon as the ward became aware that the family/patient wasn't happy with their care. This is the critical time when changes are likely to be made or when information goes missing.

- I advise complainants to tell as many people as possible and the MP is the first. Some are interested whereas others aren't, and that depends on how close their relationship is to the management. If MPs are not interested I suggest the prospective parliamentary candidate may be worth contacting, particularly nearing an election. The patient's ward County and Borough councillors should be informed too, or the parish councillor. If the hospital is an FT there will be a Governor that specifically covers the patient's ward; they should be contacted and informed of the concerns. Very often their contact details will be available on the hospital website.

- The patient's GP and the CCG need to be informed. Some are interested, others aren't – it's still very hit and miss, and that includes Healthwatch. I always advise that any letter of complaint is copied to the Secretary of State for Health and sent to their constituency address along with the Shadow Secretary and likewise to their constituency address. All of the above should be sent a copy of the letter of complaint.

- There is so much that can be done for the NHS and older people, but we are leaving it to the better organizations with better leaders to be creative but that creativity isn't being spread through the NHS for others to benefit. The problem is the poorer organizations with poor leaders are doing little to address the problems and that is leaving the elderly in those communities very poorly served.

NOTE: The use of covert surveillance in care homes may become more commonplace, as cameras can be disguised in anything from razors to radios. Many care home staff are keen on the idea too, so they can prove what great care they provide. As with all of the above, if you – as a patient, rather than a carer or worker – want to be filmed on CCTV or some hidden camera, that's your decision. But you should also have the power not to be filmed if you don't want to. Sex and masturbation can be enjoyed throughout life, and don't always have to

be filmed. Patients should know where the camera is hidden and be
able to put a towel over it for those private moments. Abusive staff
could also do the same if they find out.

Health is about freedom, and we have to balance freedom from
abuse with freedom of self-expression in private. The best way to
improve standards in care homes and in the NHS is to train, motivate
and support the staff, and to learn from the best. There are some wonderful care homes that give patients autonomy. Rooms are furnished
entirely with the patients' possessions, and this kindness and consideration extends to the careful selection of staff. In such homes, care
extends far beyond just keeping people safe to giving them meaning
and purpose in their lives and supporting them to do whatever
CLANGERS they wish. Covert surveillance would seem a horrible
intrusion. However, when care and/or trust breaks down, there may be
a case for filming to gather evidence of serious wrongdoing. With your
consent.

5

The Right Death for You

I'd really recommend listening to people when they're dying.
They have nothing to lose and so much of interest to say.
Clare, a Palliative Care Nurse

Carole's Story
For me, the fear of cancer was worse than the cancer. I've lived with it for a long time, and now I know I'm going to die from it. But I'm reasonably comfortable, I'm not in pain and I'm not frightened of it any more. My whole GP practice has been amazing, as have the Macmillan nurses, and the hospice especially really 'gets' dying. It's odd that the NHS often gets fixated on a diagnosis or trying to find a cure. But once you accept that you've tried everything you reasonably can to stay alive and you can't be cured, and you're going to die, you start concentrating on what really matters. Which is connecting with people. You start living in the moments you have before you die.

And knowing that you're dying is not a bad way to die. You have time to see all the important people in your life and tell them what you should've told them years ago. Which is how much they matter to you and how much you love them. I can't overstress the importance of doing this. So many people die without thanking those they love for a wonderful life. Most people say they'd like to go suddenly, but I'd hate to go without thanking people.

The one gift that the NHS should aim to give us all is a kind and gentle death. What distressed me most about the Mid Staffordshire scandal was that so many elderly people died in such unkind circumstances. And yet many doctors and nurses would say the most rewarding part of their jobs is helping people have gentle and kind deaths. This is much more likely to happen in a well-staffed NHS, even more so if patients are supported to die at home. We all need to plan our deaths ahead, at a place of our choosing, and think about how much intervention we would want if we are seriously ill.

You might still need drugs to take away distressing symptoms, and this too needs to be planned and they need to be ready in the house. Most doctors and nurses choose to have very little intervention when they know their time is limited. They would much rather have a gentle death at home than all the stops pulled out, and a more traumatic impersonal death, in hospital.

Have that conversation about death now. It's not always easy, but the most difficult conversations are the ones you leave until too late. You only die once, so make it a good one. I am a big fan of Dying Matters (http://dyingmatters.org), crammed full of resources for patients, relatives, carers and professionals. The NHS is fond of euphemisms – we won't say, 'What is your death wish?' – it sounds a bit Charles Bronson – but 'Have you made an Advanced Care Plan?' (ACP). The NHS website has a very good document called 'Planning Your Future Care' which everyone should read. And it gives you excellent tips about how to get into that difficult conversation. Or you could just go for it. 'Let's talk about death.'

NHS leaflets are currently being hastily rewritten because we have dropped something called the Liverpool Care Pathway, which on paper seemed a wise document to guide more people to dignified deaths. However, in the short-staffed reality of the NHS, patients and carers were not fully involved in key decisions and were not always told, say, if a medical team had decided not to call the resuscitation team in the event of a collapse. Resuscitation of older patients after cardiac or respiratory arrest is rarely successful, and I (like many doctors) would choose to die gently with the minimum of intervention. But if patients aren't involved in those decisions when they should be, it destroys the trust in a pathway that was meant to lead to a dignified death.

The best way to restore trust is for patients (i.e. all of us) to think about the options and make our death choices now – with the understanding that we can change our minds when the time comes. A home death has a lot in common with a home birth. More people want it than get it, and if you do get it you always need a Plan B. But the Plan A will only be successful with a lot of planning.

Kate Granger was an inspirational doctor with terminal cancer: she died in 2016, aged 34. She worked with elderly patients and gave this advice on death choices. 'The most important first decision is "where?" Preferred place of death is rarely achieved in the UK and I think that's because we don't plan properly. It takes a lot of effort and preparation to die at home successfully. I personally think if it is someone's wish to die at home and they have been diagnosed with an incurable condition, the planning for that event needs to start then. Patients and families need early conversations with health and social care professionals about what support and resources are available so that expectations are not dashed. Anticipatory medicines need to be in the house long before the final crisis.'

Death choices, like organ donation choices, are far more useful if you tell everyone about them. Anyone who might possibly find you on the floor one day needs to know your wishes. If you absolutely don't want to go into hospital but your neighbour with the spare key who pops in on you doesn't know that, you're likely to end up in hospital. If you don't want to be resuscitated, ask your GP to countersign an official Do Not Resuscitate form and have it on display so anyone coming to your aid can see it. The front of the fridge is a good place. If you don't have it on display, you're likely to be transferred to hospital for intensive treatment rather than cared for in your home.

WHAT'S ALL THIS THEN?

Roy and Kevin's Story

We cannot know in advance how we feel when we approach death. And we may suddenly get the urge to cling on to life as tightly as we can when we realize there may not be too much to look forward to on the other side. Some doctors fear death as much as our patients, although I'm looking forward to the lie-in when my time comes.

Dr Kevin Jones, a consultant chest physician at the Royal Bolton Hospital and superb after-dinner speaker, was frightened of dying. He cares for a lot of patients with chronic lung disease, lung cancer and mesothelioma, whose illnesses give them a slow suffocation.

And when you see patients dying and struggling for breath, it can be very distressing.

Kevin tries to take his mind off death by listening to live music at the Jolly Carter in Little Lever, Bolton. One jazz night, he was in the front row enjoying Roy Crawford, seventy, singing Elvis Presley's 'Gotta Lotta Livin' To Do'. (No, I'm not making this up.) He belted out the second verse, where he'd had 'too much living' and then collapsed and fell at Kevin's feet. He'd suffered a massive heart attack and appeared to be dead. Kevin knew the chances of resuscitating someone successfully outside hospital after a cardiac arrest were very slim. But he got someone to call 999 and gave it his best shot.

Kevin managed to bring him back to life and the paramedics arrived with a defibrillator. Roy was wheeled out of the pub conscious. This caused quite a splash in the local newspapers and Kevin, who had never successfully resuscitated somebody over seventy before, asked Roy what it was like to die. His heart had definitely stopped, and he was definitely dead until Kevin decided to save him. Did Roy remember anything? Did his whole life flash by him? Were there hounds at the gates of hell? Were there pipers at the Gates of Dawn? Did he get to meet Elvis?

Roy, amazingly, had a very clear memory of dying. He said, 'I was on stage and I remember getting into the second verse and then I thought, "Ooh, what's all this then?" And it all went black.'

So there you have it. Based on a very small, unscientific sample of one, a normal death – when medical science isn't doing all it possibly can to keep you alive, – it's a quick 'What's all this then?' and then blackout. That'll do nicely for me. But not for another thirty years.

My dad suffered from depression and took his life at thirty-nine, but others suffer the even worse tragedy of losing a child. The reason patient stories are so important in changing behaviour of medical professionals is because they help us understand what loss, hardship and courage mean, to be as good at our jobs as we can be, to work in teams that listen as well as talk, to try to spot serious illness and avoid error and harm, but above all to be kind and emotionally competent.

When I trained, I was told to leave my feelings at home and not to connect too deeply with patients, but in truth only a deeper connection between NHS staff, patients and carers can improve healthcare. It's all about building stronger relationships. I didn't truly understand chronic fatigue syndrome until I spent ninety minutes listening to the stories of each family who'd been affected. Only then did I realize what I can do to help most, how powerful every parent's instinct is to do what they can for their child and how keenly the loss is felt when we don't succeed.

Some tragedies in the NHS cannot be avoided, but there is much the NHS can do to help people make sense of their grief. Here's a stunningly good example of NHS kindness and care after a loss.

'IT WAS HUMBLING TO SEE THESE HIGHLY SKILLED PROFESSIONALS DO THEIR WORK'

Dexter's Story

Our baby Dexter was born full term weighing 8lb 6oz at the Royal Devon and Exeter Hospital. He had to be put on a ventilator straight away and was immediately transferred to the neonatal unit. Over the next few days, various investigations and tests were done which gave us hope that he could make a full recovery. But then the results of his MRI scan came through; it showed that he was severely brain-damaged due to oxygen starvation. We then made the hardest decision of our lives – to ask the doctors not to resuscitate Dexter if he was unable to breathe on his own. He was just twelve days old when he died.

Throughout this distressing time, the staff on the neonatal unit were outstanding. They treated Dexter with dignity throughout his short life and also after his life ended. We, as his parents, were cared for with kindness and compassion. No matter how many questions we had, or how many times we asked the same thing, we were given as much time as we wanted with the consultant, paediatricians or nurses. We were always treated with courtesy and respect by everyone in the unit and they did their best to accede to our wishes.

Always ensuring Dexter was as comfortable as possible, the staff made us feel that his life was as significant to them as it was to us. Nurse Jan Edwards made a print of his feet and hands and put them together in a card with some clippings of his hair. On Father's Day there was some chocolate for me that was labelled from Dexter.

As Dexter had spent his whole life in an incubator with various lines going into his little body, we asked that he be able to spend his final moments outside in the daylight. The staff arranged for us to sit outdoors in a fragrant garden with our son for his last moments. For the first time, he was not attached to lots of machines but in our arms like an ordinary baby. We cradled him in our arms as he died and then wandered over to a wooded part of the hospital grounds where we spent some time alone with him. This was important for us and the staff at the NNU did their utmost to ensure he spent his final moments in the way that we wanted.

During his time it often felt like we were powerless to help our little boy and it was humbling to see these highly skilled professionals do their work. We have the highest regard for these committed and dedicated people, who cared for our family in our moments of greatest anguish. They are an extraordinary team and a credit to the NHS.

Learning From Dexter

This book is about surviving and thriving in life, as well as the NHS, but we all must die and the NHS should help us, whenever possible, to die gently and with dignity. This in turn helps those left behind to remember and recover, and somehow make sense of it all. Life can be incredibly unkind, but healthcare without kindness is rotten. Patients and carers who are treated kindly, never forget. Those who are treated unkindly or dishonestly, rarely forgive.

When you're ill, or someone you love is ill, you may not be able to analyse your care in any depth, but you can always tell if your care is kind and you get a good sense of whether it is competent. The two often go together. Dexter's story is full of lots of small acts of thought-fulness, kindness and professionalism. The gift of chocolates on Father's Day, the prints on the card, being able to take Dexter outside into the garden, the fact that such a garden existed, the tenderness of the whole team in the face of an inevitable, heart-breaking death.

What's also significant about Dexter's care is that his father knew the names of the staff caring for him and that they felt like a team. And by giving this feedback on a public website, Patient Opinion, he is giving back to the NHS by openly thanking the team for their extraordinary care, leaving a lasting record of it, improving morale, giving others an opportunity to learn from their excellence, removing the stigma of a baby dying and highlighting to other parents who need to know that the staff on the neonatal unit at the Royal Devon and Exeter Hospital are likely to be very kind.

Doctors are human, and life can be just as unfair to us as anyone. What's extraordinary about Dr Kate Granger is that – despite her illness – she kept wanting to give back and improve the NHS to make it better for those having deeply unpleasant treatments for equally unpleasant illnesses. Doctors who actually understand what it means to be seriously ill are the wisest I know.

'I MAY ONLY HAVE A FEW MONTHS TO LIVE'

(Kate wrote this in 2014. She lived for 4 years with an incurable cancer, and died in July 2016.)

Dr Kate Granger's Story

I'm twenty-nine years old, I'm happily married to my husband Chris, I've got a very successful career as an elderly medicine registrar, I'm just two years away from fulfilling my life-long ambition of becoming a consultant in medicine for older people.

Chris and I were just starting to plan a family, we've got a lovely home in Wakefield and we were enjoying a well-deserved holiday on the California coastline. The weather was perfect and you'd think I had an idyllic life. Two days later, I was admitted to hospital in the States, acutely unwell.

The reason for my sudden illness is that I had kidney failure, and the reason for that is because my abdomen and pelvis were full of tumours. Bang. Out of the blue, age twenty-nine, I had cancer. They patched me up in the States enough to get me home, and then I returned to the UK and the NHS to pursue further investigations and treatments.

After numerous painful procedures and further scans, it was determined that I had a very rare and aggressive form of sarcoma. It's called a desmoplastic small round cell tumour. Unfortunately, the cancer has spread to my liver and bones, and I was therefore in an incurable palliative situation.

I underwent five rounds of intensive palliative chemotherapy which were complicated by serious infections, bleeding and other complications. And on New Year's Eve 2011, I made a big decision. Chris and I celebrated that day, ten years being together as a couple. We did that in hospital. The nurses made it very nice for us, we had a table, dinner, music, dimmed lights, and I even had a glass of wine, probably against the hospital rules.

But when Chris went home later that evening, I had a blood transfusion. And as that blood dripped into my poor, ravaged body I looked out over the Leeds city skyline and watched the fireworks go off and I made a decision that I'd had enough really. And that the burden of treatment was starting to outweigh the benefit. So I decided to stop.

Three weeks later, I was back on the wards, doing what I love to do, which is looking after older people. I wanted to do that job since I was a little girl. There then followed an unexpected period of stability. I was well for about twenty months, which was really unexpected because my cancer has a dismal prognosis. Most people are dead within fourteen months. But unfortunately, in October last year, my cancer started to progress again and I became very unwell, very quickly. And I had to make the heart-wrenching decision as to whether I went back to chemotherapy, or left it there and did my dying at that point.

My oncologist told me I probably had eight weeks to live, although I'm not sure how he determined that. I decided, as you can see, to have the chemotherapy. And went through another four rounds. It was tough again, and I had some very serious infections. I've now been through pretty much every type of healthcare, from primary care to surgery, I've been looked after on gynaecology wards, urology awards and oncology wards. So I've got a lot of experience as a patient now, mixed in with my experiences as a doctor.

I'd like to tell you about my core values as a clinician and patient, and why they're important to me, and tell you some stories about my experiences. My first core value is communication. Everyone talks about the importance of good communication, but I've also seen first hand the harm that bad communication can do. I'm twenty-nine years old, I know I've got cancer, I think it's confined to my abdomen. I'm expecting to have an operation, and some chemotherapy and possibly a cure. I'm in a side room in an admission ward, I can hear everything that is going on outside because I'm right by the nurses' station. I'm in pain and I'm alone. And a junior doctor comes to see me to talk about the results of my MRI scan I had earlier in the week. I've never met this doctor before.

He came into my room, sat down in the chair next to me and looked away from me. Without any warning shot or checking my baseline understanding, or asking if I wanted anybody with me, he just said to me simply, 'Your cancer has spread.' He then couldn't leave the room quick enough, and I was left in deep psychological distress with the nurses not knowing what he told me, and I never saw him again.

I think I'm a little bit psychologically scarred by that experience although I wouldn't like to admit it. We break bad news in the NHS every single day, it's going on as we speak. But when we do it we need to consider how we leave the patient and how they have to live that story. In contrast, when my oncologist told me my final diagnosis, I had a much better experience. I'd got to know him over the few preceding weeks. He asked me if I wanted somebody with me at that particular point, but I didn't. He gently sat down beside me, actually on my hospital bed, against the rules. He held my hand and gently told me my diagnosis. He then sat in silence, and let me take that in, and supported me through the eventual emotional breakdown that followed. That experience, although probably more devastating news, wasn't as distressing for me as the first experience.

My second core value as a clinician is about the little things. I really think the little things matter when you're a patient, and they're what can make the difference between a good experience and a bad experience. When I say the little things, I mean somebody holding your hand, somebody introducing themselves and somebody sitting down next to you instead of standing over you. I mean someone taking that extra moment to really listen to your fears and anxieties.

I was very sick a couple of months ago, probably the sickest I've been on my journey. It was a Saturday night, and the on-call oncologist came to see me. And besides all the other things he did for me, including phoning the on-call urologist, talking to the radiology doctors, talking to the microbiology doctors, changing all my treatments round, the one thing he did was kneel down beside my bed, put his hand on my arm gently, and say, 'Kate, you're going to be okay.'

Because he'd recognized how frightened and vulnerable I was feeling in that situation. A few days later in that admission a registrar came to see me and she wanted to talk to me about the positive blood culture results I just received. It was very scary for me to have a bacteraemia. And she refused to sit down when I asked her to take a seat on the chair that was right next to my bed. She thought I was asking her for her benefit, but I wasn't. I was asking her for my benefit so that we could have a conversation on the same level. Instead she stood looming over me, making me feel little and less in control. Those little things do really matter and everyone can do them.

My third core value is person-centred care. In January I was admitted to hospital with febrile neutropenia. At the time, I was put on the standard antibiotic protocol, given some intravenous fluids, reviewed by the consultant and transferred to another ward. On that ward, a nurse came to give me my antibiotics at lunchtime. The drugs had been changed from the standard protocol to those used for much more serious infections. I didn't know anything about this change in antibiotics. The first thought that went through my head was, has she got the right drug chart? Or had somebody made a prescribing error? My second thought was, oh my god they've got the really strong stuff out like Domestos, I must have something

really serious. Looking back through the medical notes, I realized
what had happened. The consultant oncologist had reviewed me,
he'd been very diligent and looked at all my microbiology results
on the computer, he'd found that I'd grown a multi-resistant E. coli
from my urine infection a couple of weeks earlier, and correctly
advised the junior doctor, after phoning a microbiologist, to do
some more tests. The junior doctor had done these, she phoned the
microbiologist and clearly documented this in the medical notes
and changed my antibiotics appropriately.

That was an episode of safe care, I received the right treatment, in
a timely fashion, but it forgot one thing, perhaps the most important
thing. Me. I wish it could be written across my notes in big bold
letters that I want to know absolutely everything. This was a serious
change of treatment that they'd forgotten to tell me. I think that
something like that just happens. I've done it as a junior doctor. You
take your jobs list and you're so ingrained in having all these jobs to
do that you get stuck in the system and you forget the patient.

My first job was in Dewsbury Hospital, working for Dr Kemp. He
was a diabetologist, and a very wise clinician coming towards the end
of his career. He took me under his wing, because he knew I wanted
to become a physician. And he said to me one day, 'Kate, being a
physician is about painting a picture. It's not about ticking a box or
following a protocol. And during the admission, you're painting extra
bits of the picture every day until you've got the full painting.'

My fourth core value is to see me and not just my disease. I've
been referred to, within earshot, by several consultants as that girl
with DSRCT. Within one sentence, I'm just reduced to somebody
with a rare cancer, and nothing else. At a vulnerable time in my life,
when I was feeling pretty low emotionally anyway, that's not
something that I want to hear. I'm much more than just a rare cancer,
I'm a wife, a daughter, a doctor, an auntie to a new baby in a few
months. I like to play the flute, I'm an avid baker, and there are lots
and lots of things about me that are more important.

And this has become something that's very important to me in my
clinical practice since my return to work after my diagnosis. I want to
know more about my patients so I can contextualize their disease

within their own lives. And that's extremely important for what I do as a physician to the elderly. People have got loads of stories to tell you about their lives. I've looked after a gentleman who was an Olympic cyclist in his day. And people have written him off as being too frail to treat. But actually, when you asked this gentleman, he'd been walking up mountains the week before he got ill with pneumonia. So I fought for his ICU admission and he got better and got out of hospital.

I sent this tweet a few months ago when I was on a urology ward. Everyone from the healthcare assistant, housekeeper and nurse kept on referring to me as bed seven. It was even 'Bed seven, what would you like to drink?' My name is Kate. Coming into hospital is an extremely dehumanizing experience. You really do leave your personality and humanity on the doorstep, and sometimes even your dignity. At least keeping your name is one thing we can all do to re-humanize the experience and not reduce people to numbers or diseases.

I took a selfie of me looking really knackered in hospital when I had really been through the routine: 2am obs; 4am change your intravenous fluids; 6am obs again; 6:30am, just as you're getting back to sleep, antibiotics; 8am obs. And so it goes on. Every night. By day three, I was extremely sleep deprived. I was getting very ratty and I just wanted to rest. All I wanted to do was to just sleep. I'd been very unwell. And so the interruptions started. A phlebotomist woke me up to take my blood but I'd already had my blood taken from my portacath earlier that morning.

Then a healthcare assistant came to change my bed. Could that not have waited just a few hours while I caught up on my sleep? Then somebody came to offer me a tea or coffee. I've been on this ward multiple times. I don't drink tea or coffee. The straw that broke the camel's back was the cleaner who yelled at me until I was awake, to ask if he could clean my room. At that point I turned my sheet over my head, turned my back on the world and tried to forget where I was. I self-discharged later that day, probably against medical advice. I went home, had sixteen hours sleep, and felt a lot better for it.

In August, I was having a routine operation to replace the stents that drain my kidneys. That surgery was uncomplicated, and I have a surgeon I have absolute trust in. He is an amazing man. I went home four hours after I had my anaesthetic, as soon as I got my final set of obs. Unfortunately, thirty-six hours later I was back in the emergency department with a high fever, and a low blood pressure. A serious post-op infection.

I was triaged by a nurse who I'd worked with in the past and was lovely to me. And then things started to slide. I was clerked in by a surgical doctor who had no name and no role. So I asked him, and he seemed a little bit put out that I wanted to know what grade of doctor he was and what his name was. Then I assume a healthcare support worker or a healthcare assistant came to cannulate me and take my bloods. She had no name.

Then a nurse came to give me my antibiotics. She had no name either. And finally, somebody introduced themselves to me, and that was a porter. And this porter was called Brian. Brian was a little star, he helped me get onto his trolley, he fetched extra pillows and blankets, he noticed I was in pain and took extra care to push me over the bumps in the corridors, and all the time he was talking reassuringly to my husband and me. He was exhibiting the little things. And in doing so, he relieved so many anxieties.

There then followed a week-long admission to surgical ward, where the lack of introduction seemed to permeate through every professional group, and all the support staff. When somebody did introduce themselves, it made such a difference. You knew which nurse to ask for, it started a human connection. So one evening I was moaning to my husband about this. Chris is a logistics manager for a big supermarket. He is a very practical person and he told me to stop whingeing and do something about it. And the result of that conversation was #hello my name is.

This is a social media campaign that encourages anybody who has a patient-facing role to introduce themselves to their patients. I believe it's much more than common courtesy. I believe it's about a human connection. It's about beginning a therapeutic relationship, about building trust and rapport. And as a patient, you are really bottom of the pile in the power stakes. As a health professional, you have so much detailed knowledge about the people you're looking after. And one way of rebalancing those scales of power is by introducing yourself, asking what a patient would like to be called and explaining what you're going to do. These are really important little things that take no time and cost no money.

I wrote a blog about #hello my name is and hundreds of people got involved in the campaign and started tweeting about it. It became clear that my experience was not unique. And people were having the same experience throughout health and social care. People took this to heart, it seemed to strike a chord. There were posters, there were ward introduction boards, there were lanyards, there were simple reminders in the workplace, there were screensavers, it permeated through healthcare conferences and magazines, there were selfie campaigns, you name it and people have done it.

The government has heard of it as well. If you turn to page thirty-six of the response to the Francis inquiry, you'll find a box all about '#hello my name is'. Jeremy Hunt mentioned it in a speech about continuity of care and treating patients as people. He didn't actually ask my permission to use the idea. We presented it at the NHS Expo in March and I took it to Paris to the International Health Care Forum, and I indoctrinated one of my healthcare heroes, Don Berwick. If you look at the social media analytics, it's had a massive impact, after only ten months. According to Simpler, there have been over twenty-six million Twitter impressions. Fifteen thousand people have tweeted about it. I want to go on tour around the NHS.

I would love one of my legacies to be an NHS that considers patients as people, and really considers the whole person. I only probably have a few months to live, but I'm determined to use some of the energy I have left in a productive way, to improve the quality of care we deliver to patients in the NHS.

Kate's advice for anyone with a serious illness negotiating the NHS:

- Ask for a copy of all your letters.

- Do not let anything be written about you that you have not seen yourself.

- Make sure you understand what is happening to you.

- Ask, ask, ask.

- Be involved in decision-making and don't let things just happen to you passively.

- Take an active role in your care.

- Be part of the team looking after you.

- Keep a little diary of major events in your illness. It allows you to give a rapid history to anyone that sees you with all the info they will need.

- Keep a list of your medicines with you.

- Information is power, especially in the healthcare setting.

- The power balance is very much in favour of the NHS and its staff, but active patients can redress this.

For more about Kate's inspirational legacy and campaign for compassionate cure, go to www.hellomynameis.org.uk.

LIFE AFTER A DEATH

We all have to experience grief at some time and we all cope in our own way. When my father died, I was seven but I coped – then and now – by thinking, what would my Dad want for me? I knew he would want me to get the most from my one wild, short and precious life. I love the story below, because it shows a wonderful man caring for his wife, coming to terms with her death and learning that life must go on. Recovering after loss is fundamental to surviving life and the NHS.

'I DIDN'T REALLY NEED TO FEEL ALL THAT GUILTY'

Bert's Story
My wife had multi infarct dementia and when she came towards what I've since realized was the end, she stopped eating and

drinking. I then had these difficult decisions to make and I was obsessed. Okay, I was still going out to dance because you have to have diversions, if you don't have diversions you would go mad yourself.

But every day I had to run over the decision about whether we were doing the right thing. I used to say when I got to the home: 'Have you tried her with food today? How did she get on?' 'She had a yoghurt and half a spoonful of custard,' and so on. That was a tremendous turning point because the guilt then was different. Am I condemning her to die by taking this attitude? And then having to reconcile the guilt with the fact that when I was out dancing I was really enjoying myself. Obviously, I couldn't inflict that on other people. I don't know whether that requires a split personality but I suppose I really had one.

But the interesting thing about the final turning point, which of course on her death was just that, after the initial emotional impact, was the tremendous relief that it brought. Again, that was something that made me feel slightly guilty but I had to reconcile my feeling of guilt, I had to balance it with the fact that it was so much better for her. She'd stopped suffering, she'd gone peacefully, she'd gone without pain, I'd done my best so really I didn't really need to feel all that guilty.

And I must say that, although I wouldn't have believed it at the time and perhaps for some two or three months afterwards, I now find myself talking to my wife, or to her photograph, as though she were still here. But talking without any inhibitions at all, without any feelings of guilt. So that was a tremendous turning point really. Whatever has happened to her since she died it's certainly made a big difference from my point of view. And we're still good mates.

There are many other insightful and moving stories on the healthtalk.org website – my favourite health website. It simply uses the experiences of patients and carers in the NHS to help and guide others confronting the same illnesses and situations. I tell medical students and doctors to use it too. If empathy can be taught, it will be from patient stories.

GOING OUT IN STYLE: MAKING
DEATH EARN ITS LIVING

> When you've got cancer, you notice one or two little odd things
> which other people don't, one of which is the sudden proliferation
> round the house of skewers and knitting needles and cork-screws,
> sometimes covered in blood, sometimes not . . . because you've
> been trying to pierce new holes in your old belts.
>
> **Miles Kington, 1941–2008**

So observed the late humorist Miles Kington in his final book, *How Shall I tell the Dog?*, an object lesson in how to die with style and humour, and 'how to make cancer work for its living'.

Miles died of pancreatic cancer at the age of sixty-six. He was a great friend and an inspiration in life and death. He launched the comedy career of Struck Off and Die in 1990 (with a very favourable review), showed me how to play petanque (with a little alcohol on board) and taught me the secret of comedy. Most jokes have a punch-line you can see coming for miles, but the best jokes take you somewhere completely unexpected. Hence the belt holes.

Miles was one of our most prolific humorists, writing a daily column for thirty years, first for *The Times*, and then for *The Independent*. Prior to that, he was on the staff of *Punch*, where he started the popular 'Let's Parler Franglais' column, 'which furnished four Penguin paperbacks and many middle class loos'. His own loo was stuffed with books, as was the rest of his idyllic house near Bath. He'd write a column, share it with his wife Caroline, bake some bread, argue about the shape of the loaf, cycle to Bradford on Avon, buy some rare jazz records, stop and chat, think about tomorrow's column and amble home. He really knew how to do the best CLANGERS. Then he started losing weight.

> In my trim days, my waist was a good, elegant thirty-two inches, but
> when I started to enjoy food more and take less exercise, it gradually
> crept up to thirty-six inches, nudging thirty-seven inches . . . Now I'm

down to thirty-two inches again. However, it's not a slim elegant thirty-two inches any more. It is a scrawny, puckered-navel kind of thinness which means that having tightened my belts progressively, I have now come to the last hole provided and beyond. Making a new hole is easier said than done . . . Hence the abandoned tools all over the place. And the blood marks.

How Shall I Tell the Dog? takes the form of a series of letters from Miles to his friend and literary agent Gill Coleridge. The title is taken from a musing on the delicate subject of not outliving your pets, and how to break the news. The scope of topics covered is vast and entirely unpredictable, as you'd expect from a humorist whose brain keeps changing direction in the comedic equivalent of a knight's move. There are outrageous suggestions for marketing your cancer (board games, funeral videos, tie-in books) and some funny yet moving observations on the language of cancer, the power of self-pity, who to trust and whether someone will invent a test for 'the will to live'. And there are conversations with doctors, my favourite of which is an oncologist soliciting advice on how to get his own book published.

Some of which should be taken with a pinch of salt. Another of Miles' comedic tips was that 'any writer worth his salt improves the story until it's worth telling'. These letters contain truths that have been polished into pearls. I had lunch with Miles shortly after he'd discovered his diagnosis, and he was already thinking of a book. 'How many stages does pancreatic cancer have?' 'What do you mean by stages?' 'Well, chapters.' Miles coped by disappearing inside his head: 'The best time to joke about death is when you never think you're going to die.' He used to start letters that he'd taken far too long to respond to with: 'Dear so-and-so, While sorting out my papers prior to my death, I came across a letter from you which . . .' This is only funny if you're not going to die imminently. But Miles really did have papers to sort out. And he thought it would make a fine documentary, facing up not just to the great void beyond, but 'the twenty years of accumulation on the desk, and indeed on the carpet around the desk'. The task would take up a whole programme. 'Miles Kington clears his desk and dies.'

Miles never did get round to clearing his desk, but he carried on writing until he was just too knackered, then crawled into his bed and died peacefully at home. His last column appeared in *The Independent* on the day he died. His editor had no idea he was ill. Writing is a great way of teaching us empathy, but very few books can give you the courage to taunt death. *How Shall I Tell the Dog?* is one of them. When my time comes, I'll get this book out and turn to 'Infrequently Asked Questions'. 'Can the experience of dying from cancer be included in the Duke of Edinburgh award scheme?' There's no reason why smiling and death can't be bedfellows.

I'm all for assertive, active, engaged, included, informed patients – and I might even be one when my time comes. But health is ultimately about freedom, and the ultimate freedom is to die gently at home.

POSTSCRIPT – Stan and My Story

My wonderful step-father Stan, was diagnosed with (very probable) pancreatic cancer in 2014. I say very probable, because he decided not to have a biopsy for reasons that will become apparent. But his CT scan showed a mass at the head of the pancreas which was almost certainly cancer.

The pancreas, like the ovaries, is hidden away and so cancer there often presents late. Often it's only when the cancer presses on the bile duct and causes obstructive jaundice that it makes itself known. Dark urine, pale stools and yellow skin and eyes are hard to ignore. Stan was scanned quickly and kindly in our local NHS hospital in Bath, and a stent was put in to unblock the bile duct and relieve his jaundice. This all happened within a week, and again the staff were compassionate, competent and good communicators.

The next thing I did was to wise up on pancreatic cancer. I read the book, *Fast Facts – diseases of the pancreas and biliary tract*. I find these books incredibly useful as a way of getting up to speed quickly on any disease, and I recommend them to patients. I also explored pancreatic cancer charity websites, the NICE website and the wonderful healthtalk.org website which has very useful films, stories and experiences from patients and carers about how the disease progresses and what the risks and benefits of treatment are. The best chance of cure is surgery, but sadly:

- 45 per cent of patients have metastases at diagnosis.

- 40 per cent of patients do not have distant metastases but have locally advanced inoperable disease.

- Only 15 per cent have localized, non-metastatic potentially resectable (remove it by surgery) disease.

Overall the survival rate for pancreatic at five years is only 4–5 per cent. We don't hear much about this in the press because most of the people who get it aren't alive to tell their stories. Even with surgery, the five-year survival is just 25 per cent for 'node negative' patients (i.e. the cancer hasn't spread to surrounding lymph nodes), and 10 per cent for 'node positive' patients. Even in operable cases, the majority of patients still die of the disease. However, if the tumour has not spread at all, and you survive surgery and get through chemotherapy too, your chance of being alive at five years is 29 per cent. Still not great, but a lot better than 5 per cent.

On the downside, surgery for pancreatic cancer is one of the biggest operations there is, takes a long time to recover from, has very unpleasant side effects and is one hell of a challenge even for a younger person. Stan is eighty-four. If you're even considering it, you need to go to a specialist unit – a large centre that does lots of the operations and can show that they do them well.

So where do you find out the best place to have pancreatic cancer surgery in the NHS? One of the authors of the Fast Facts book is John Neoptolemos, a professor of surgery in Liverpool. The pancreatic cancer section of his hospital website (www.rlbuht.nhs.uk) was extremely useful in terms of what to expect (the process) but there was no information on outcomes.

The NHS Choices website, and the new My Cancer Treatment and My NHS websites were equally devoid of outcomes to compare different specialist centres for pancreatic cancer. The NHS Choices website was very good on the disease and treatment options, but ridiculously inaccurate and confusing when I searched for hospital pancreatic cancer services near my postcode, citing day hospitals, care homes and nurseries.

I know the private data company Doctor Foster Intelligence (DFI) does collect the comparative death rates at thirty days for all sorts of operations, but again, searching its website drew a blank. I know people who work for DFI and I could easily make a phone call and get the data but I wanted to try as someone who doesn't have privileged contacts. I typed 'pancreatic cancer surgery NHS mortality rate' into Google and the fourth hit was Imperial College Healthcare NHS Trust in London. It celebrated its own outcomes and published graphs from DFI: 'The two graphs linked below demonstrate that Imperial College Healthcare NHS Trust has the best UK surgical outcomes in both pancreatic and liver surgery. There was zero mortality in patients undergoing either pancreatic or liver surgery in the last two years and ICHNT recorded the highest three year survival rates for pancreatic cancer in the UK.'

What it meant by 'zero mortality' was that all its patients were alive thirty days after surgery. Cambridge and Liverpool also had very low mortality rates, and if I was able to choose I would opt for Liverpool because it does by far the largest number of operations of the three. My nearest specialist unit also did a large number of cases but had a higher mortality rate.

Even if you manage to track down data that points you to one of the best services in the NHS, you may not be willing or able to travel a large distance to another unit, and you may prefer to go to your local unit. And even if you'd travel the world and back for your loved one, a cash-strapped NHS is trying to restrict 'out of area' referrals in many parts of the UK, even though the NHS Constitution gives you the right to choose. Just as you may be denied a drug you think you need towards the end of life, you may also be denied a specialist service you have carefully researched and chosen because the NHS sometimes resists free movement around the system.

As I was pondering this, a surgeon friend of mine said that he knew Professor Neoptolemos in Liverpool, and he would be happy to talk through the options on the phone. This is clearly not an option open to everyone but I wanted to find out the oldest patients he had operated successfully on, and whether patients found it easy to get a referral to his unit if they lived a long way from Liverpool. He said he often operated on fit patients in their eighties who had done well, and that many patients came from outside his area because they wanted to be treated in a specialist centre with huge expertise and cutting-edge research.

His passion for improving pancreatic surgery services and outcomes was inspirational, but it's Stan's cancer and he wasn't keen on such major surgery at eighty-four. He'd had heart surgery in Bristol thirteen years previously and made a brilliant recovery but the odds then were much better. We saw a very kind consultant called Terry Farrant in Bath, who showed us the CT scan and said that, although the liver was clear, the cancer had spread to the lymph nodes. Surgery, if it ever had been an option, wasn't now. He offered to arrange a biopsy – which would have meant another endoscopy – to name the tumour. It might be a lymphoma rather than an adenocarcinoma, which might respond better to chemotherapy. But Stan had looked at the same websites I had, thought and talked through the options and decided he didn't think the benefits of chemotherapy were worth the side effects. As for naming the cancer, we decided on Delores.

I then expected Stan to be discharged from the upper GI cancer service to the GP, district nurse and palliative care team. But Dr Farrant said he'd like to keep in touch with Stan, to see how this 'watchful waiting' went, and that the clinical nurse specialist would be in touch. If he needed help, advice, pancreatic supplements or another stent in future it could easily be arranged. Stan was left feeling that he'd made the right decision but was still connected to the team that had been so kind to him.

Stan had six months free from jaundice and feeling well. He stopped all his heart medications, ate for England and actually put weight on to start with. He saw all his friends and family, shared fantastic stories and was surrounded by love. For his last Christmas, he was able to walk up Burledge hill, eat a huge portion of turkey and pudding, and enjoy a couple of glasses of wine. He planned to die at home and we wanted to support him.

After six months, Stan's stent blocked up, he became jaundiced again and it was too painful for him to eat. We had a hospital bed installed at home and a wonderful team comprising of my extraordinary mum, district nurses, his GP, the palliative care team, a carer and the out of hours team. They all new that he didn't want to be resuscitated and took great care to control his symptoms so he wasn't in distress or pain. Stan had the best legal death he could have had in the UK.

But I think it could have been better. Stan hoped he would die quickly from his pancreatic cancer but he slowly and inexorably wasted away. From the moment he could no longer eat, it took a month for him to die. He was not in any physical distress, but he did not want us to see him wasting away and that caused him anguish. He wanted me to assist his death and, had it been legal, it would have been the kindest thing to do and I would gladly have helped. When he finally died, in May 2015, he was the shell of the Stan I knew.

If we are to control our health, I think we should also be able to have some control over our death. Stan's death taught me that, even with the best palliative care in the world, many people would choose to die earlier. I do not want anyone to see me wasting away to a husk. I have become a patron of My Death, My Decision (www.mydeath-mydecision.org.uk), to support a change in the law on assisted dying.

FURTHER CLANGING

*'Time is the substance I am made of. Time is a river which
sweeps me along, but I am the river; it is a tiger which destroys me,
but I am the tiger; it is a fire which consumes me, but I am the fire.'*
Jorge Luis Borges

Time is limited for all of us, but the things we can do with our time are
limitless. Great art and literature can give you far more insight, meaning and wisdom than any number of self-help books, so choose wisely.
In essence, health means being well enough to do what you want to
do, and be who you want to be. Most lives need living, not medicaliz-
ing. And for 90 per cent of symptoms, you're better off with a dog than
a doctor. Over half of all symptoms are 'medically unexplained'. Most
get better with time and compassion, others never go but improve with
acceptance and diversion. The trick is to spot the 10 per cent that can't
be licked better.

Some serious illnesses can be delayed or even prevented by living
well and early diagnosis, but others simply come down to bad luck.
They are caused by life circumstances, genetic predispositions or mutations that you may not be able to do anything about. So don't beat
yourself up about it. Blame and guilt waste energy that could be spent
on living. When you're seriously ill, you may just want to be cared for
rather than get involved in your care. However, as you get stronger and
braver, the chances are you'll be able to contribute to your recovery
and improve your life by doing your daily CLANGERS.

To get the best from life and the NHS, think CLANG – CONNECT,
laugh and build good relationships with the people treating and caring
for you, LEARN as much about your illness, the choices available to
you and the care you should be getting, and be as ACTIVE as you can,
both as a partner in your healthcare and with the NHS, and in living

and staying well outside the NHS. You need to NOTICE what is happening in your body, observe your treatment and speak up if you have any concerns or questions. And you need to GIVE BACK to those caring for and treating you, to the NHS and to other patients so they can benefit from what you've experienced and learned. To have the energy to do this, you also need to EAT WELL, RELAX and SLEEP – three things that aren't always synonymous with hospital care.

Often, what you can do for yourself and with the help of your community to improve your life and health far outweighs what the NHS can do for you. The website www.community-shop.co.uk is a brilliant example. Where I live, wellbeingoptions.co.uk will signpost you to a treasure trove of community activity and support.

GETTING YOUR HEAD TOGETHER

It's very hard to have a healthy body without a healthy mind. *Mindfulness – A Practical Guide to Finding Peace in a Frantic World* by Mark Williams and Danny Penman can work well for stress, anxiety, unhappiness and exhaustion. *Mindfulness for Health: A Practical Guide to Relieving Pain, Reducing Stress and Restoring Wellbeing* by Vidyamala Burch and Danny Penman is also very good. You can get a free taster on www.franticworld.com and www.bemindful.co.uk. These strategies use a very simple form of meditation that has been proven to work, and in Ruby Wax's *Sane New World* you get them with added humour.

Positive psychology also has a good evidence base for improving your life. A useful website is www.positivepsychologytraining.co.uk, run by Miriam Akhtar, the author of *Positive Psychology for Overcoming Depression*. The book *Thrive: The Power of Evidence-Based Psychological Therapies* by Richard Layard and David Clark is a useful summary of which therapies work and for whom. Getting access to them in the NHS is sadly not always easy: www.iapt.nhs.uk may link to psychological services near you. The website www.actionforhappiness.org has a great philosophy and good advice for those seeking to increase happiness and reduce misery not just in themselves but in those around them.

Giving back to others is crucial for your emotional health, and the

NHS and social care system needs all the volunteers it can get. A good place to start is your local NHS services or www.royalvoluntaryservice. org.uk, www.dementiafriends.org.uk, www.kissingitbetter.co.uk and www.thesilverline.org.uk.

The website www.connectingwithpeople.org has been written by very compassionate professionals and service users who have struggled with the thought that life is not worth living. It gives good advice on staying safe, holding off suicidal thoughts and getting help. In addition, www.samaritans.org, www.sane.org.uk, www.childline.org.uk and www.thesilverline.org.uk are also great sources of support.

GETTING YOUR HEAD AROUND HEALTH

'We do not own the land, the land owns us. But we belong to it. The completeness of being who you are, where you are, is a really good feeling.'

Bob Randall, Aboriginal elder
www.globalonenessproject.org

Medicine, and the NHS, has much too narrow a focus. We fight disease within four walls when the possibilities of health stretch from horizon to horizon. The limits of medicine are vastly outweighed by the limitless ways we can live well with compassion, value and purpose. Two great books to help you explore the possibilities of living a healthier life and feeling much better for it are *Why We Sleep* by Professor Matthew Walker, and *The 4 Pillar Plan (Relax, Eat, Move, Sleep)* by Dr Ranjan Chatterjee. Both are full of CLANGERS advice. Simply by getting your sleep as good as it can be can transform your life, and give you all the energy you need to work on your CLANGERS.

GETTING YOUR HEAD AROUND SELF-CARE

Both www.nhs.uk and www.patient.co.uk have lots of free advice and apps for living well with and without illnesses, and treating self-limiting conditions. *Diagnosing Your Health Symptoms for Dummies* by Dr Knut Schroeder is a great book for learning when and how to self-care, and when and how to seek help. *Don't Die Young* by Professor Alice Roberts has some great illustrations and all the anatomy you need to know. The Student Health App is a fantastic source of reliable health information, and not just for students. St John Ambulance has an app that tells you what to do in an emergency and it runs hands-on courses to practise. The *NHS Choose Well* information tells you what you need to do for which symptoms – self-care, pharmacy, dial 111, see your GP, walk-in centre or 999/emergency department. All this information should be on your GP practice website and as a leaflet in the surgery.

GETTING YOUR HEAD AROUND THE EVIDENCE

Know Your Chances by Steven Woloshin, Lisa Schwartz and Gilbert Welch is a great book, available free, to help you understand the trade-offs between different tests and treatments. The www.testingtreatments.org website tells you how treatments are tested, and why these tests should be (but aren't always) fair and reliable, while www.senseaboutscience.org and www.askforevidence.org encourages you to ask for the evidence behind screening and treatment choices and helps you make sense of it. A great book on the limits of medicine, the perils of over-treating and the import-ance of evidence is *The Patient Paradox* by Dr Margaret McCartney. *Bad Science* and *Bad Pharma* by Ben Goldacre will make you more questioning and sceptical of the claims made about all health interventions, and help you understand the vested interests. The site www.alltrials.net is a power-ful campaign trying to ensure all the data and results of all clinical trials for drugs and devices currently in use are in the public domain. This move to 'open data' would allow more scrutiny, improve trust in the drug industry and lessen error, bias and wrongdoing.

Remember, five different doctors may give you five different opinions or even diagnoses. We don't do it deliberately, we just have the same problems getting to grips with the evidence that you do. Which is why it's always good to ask what the evidence is for a particular diagnosis or opin-ion, make a note of it, check it out on, say, the www.nice.org.uk website and then challenge it politely if you have any questions. Often, evidence is lacking and you have to work as a team to make 'a best guess'.

Drugs Without the Hot Air – Minimising the harms of legal and illegal drugs by David Nutt is well written, evidence-based and does exactly what it says on the cover. The website www.rxisk.org helps you weigh up the benefits and side effects of legal drugs, and take them safely. If you want to know the science behind the bold or scary claims of newspaper headlines, then the NHS Behind the Headlines site is a great way of understanding both how the media and how science works: www.nhs.uk/news.

A good summary of the evidence that involved patients get better NHS care *and* can also make the NHS better is found in *Engaging Patients in Healthcare* by Angela Coulter. Patient engagement is a huge untapped resource in the NHS but you may need help and support to wade through the complex choices you face.

The NHS itself has had fifteen reorganizations in the thirty years I've worked in it, but evidence as to whether any of them have worked is woefully lacking. Like a new treatment, reorganizations need to be properly tested before they're forced on the NHS and patients. Some politicians have a nasty habit of confusing evidence with ideology and vested interest, risking lives, money and the mental health of NHS staff and patients in the process. Politicians on all sides must collaborate to build a better, joined-up NHS and social care system based on fairness, compassion, the best evidence and value for our money.

GETTING YOUR OWN DATA

If you want to, you should be able to read anything written about you in the NHS. Consider getting copies of your medical records, investigation results and all letters written about you. Search www.nhs.uk to find out how. Read and discuss them with friends, family and clinical staff. Ask to see entries as they are typed in at each consultation. Speak up if you don't understand anything written about you or (as often happens) you spot errors in your records. If you don't correct them, they may well be repeated and magnified. The NHS has been promising to provide you with online access to your medical records via an NHS app for many years. The site www.patientsknowbest.com is leading the way in giving patients more control of their healthcare, in partnership with the staff treating them.

GETTING YOUR HEAD AROUND YOUR SYMPTOMS

Most symptoms get better in time, so how do you spot those that won't? It's an ever-present dilemma for NHS staff, patients and carers. The www.nice.org.uk has very useful referral guidelines for suspected cancer and feverish illness in children, and www.macmillan.org.uk also has good advice and decision support for spotting cancer. Life-threatening illnesses are often sudden and severe, but not always. The NHS website and patient.co.uk have symptom sorters to guide you. If you're worried, and can't easily speak to a GP, phone 111. For choking, chest pain, suspected stroke, suspected meningitis, blackouts, severe blood loss, breathing difficulties and overdoses, phone 999. Even the best and most experienced doctors don't always get these calls right, and neither will you.

GETTING YOUR HEAD AROUND A CONSULTATION

SCAN your problems in advance – what are your Symptoms and Story? What are your Concerns? What is your Assessment? What are your Needs?

Arrive in good time for your appointment. If you're anxious, breathe deeply and slowly, and concentrate on the air going in and out of your lungs.

Take a copy of your SCAN and CLANG during the consultation. Ask three good questions, e.g.:

- 'What else could it be?', 'How would I know?' and 'What should I do if it doesn't get better?'

- 'What is my main problem?', 'What do I need to do now?' and 'Why is it important for me to do this?'

- 'What are my options?', 'What are the pros and cons of each option?' and 'How do I get support to help me make a decision that is right for me?'

Usually you have time to mull over a complicated choice, share it with friends and family and do some research. Don't rush it. And always ask 'What is most likely to happen if we just watch and wait?'

Take notes and leave with a clear action plan and safety net (Plan B).

GETTING YOUR HEAD AROUND AN ILLNESS

The websites www.nhs.uk, www.healthtalk.org and www.patient.co.uk will give you a wealth of reliable information and an understanding of your condition, the treatment options and trade-offs, and what to expect. A good charity website and helpline are life-savers when you fall into the river of illness. The specialist centres for your condition often have close links for support and research to the best charities. The *Fast Facts* series of books can quickly get you up to speed about any condition if you want a higher level of knowledge – www.fastfacts. com. You should have an NHS care plan for long-standing illnesses, and simple texting services such as Flo help you manage them much better. The websites www.embarrassingproblems.com and www.channel4embarrassingillnesses.com give you the facts and courage to seek help when you're embarrassed. Other patients and carers are often the most useful sources of information.

There are lots of great books and blogs written about the experience and meaning of being ill. *Illness: the Cry of the Flesh* by Havi Carel is wonderful, as is *I Think There's Something Wrong with Me* by Nigel Smith. *My Baglady Life* is a great campaigning blog by Wendy Lee. *Surviving and Thriving – My Encounter with Brain Cancer* by David Grant is available via www.lulu.com. *What the F*** is Normal?* by Francesca Martinez is a moving and funny memoir about finding your own path in life.

GETTING YOUR HEAD AROUND CHOICE

Ultimately, medicine is about choosing wisely under pressure: human beings in imperfect systems struggling to do the right thing with limited time and resources. Medicine itself has limits (we're all going to die), and often the wisest choice may be to watch, wait, love and support. Many choices are complicated trade-offs between risks and benefits. Your need to understand the science and know what matters to you most to choose wisely. There's a great website, www.choosingwisely. co.uk, that lists the trade-offs for an increasing number of treatments. It advises you to think BRAN whenever you discuss and share a treatment decision with a doctor or nurse:

1. What are the *B*enefits?

2. What are the *R*isks?

3. What are the *A*lternatives?

4. What if I do *N*othing?

And there are some great decision aids at decionaid.ohri.ca. The www. nice.org.uk site is where to go to find out what treatment choices you are entitled to in the NHS, and to what standard. If you can't get a treatment you think you're entitled to, get the support of NHS staff, a good charity and even the media to challenge the decision.

Deciding *where* to have your treatment is harder, because reliable comparative data in the NHS for most specialties is in its infancy, and even if you decide you want to travel to a specialist centre outside your area, you may struggle to get funding for it. The Care Quality Commission in England (www.cqc.org.uk) aims to tell you which NHS and private medical, social and dental services are providing the required services to the required standard – like the rest of the NHS, it sometimes makes mistakes. The websites www.patientopinion.org.uk and www.iwantgreatcare. org give feedback on services from a patient's perspective. It's too early to say how useful the new My Cancer Treatment (www.mycancertreatment.

nhs.uk) and My NHS (www.nhs.uk/mynhs) websites are for guiding wise choices about where to get treatment but they're worth trying, if only to give feedback as to what information you need. The NHS is way ahead of most other health systems in the openness of its data.

GETTING YOUR HEAD AROUND AGEING

Despite the bad press, there has never been a better time to age. Older people are happier, healthier and – yes – older than we ever have been. Age UK has a wealth of information and support. *How to Age Positively* by Guy Roberson is a neat little evidence-based book that might make you feel more optimistic about ageing.

GETTING YOUR HEAD AROUND DEATH

No-one gets out of here alive, as Jim Morrison observed. We're all slowly rusting to death and returning to room temperature. But a good life should end with a gentle death. *Being Mortal* by Atul Gwande, *The Other Side* and *The Bright Side* by Kate Granger, *With the End in Mind* by Kathryn Mannix and *Living with Dying* by Margaret McCartney should put you in the mood. The website www.dyingmatters.org helps you plan well in advance. *How Shall I Tell the Dog?* by Miles Kington helps you laugh in advance. If you want to explore assisted dying, try *I'll See Myself Out, Thank You* by Colin Brewer and Michael Irwin.

GETTING YOUR HEAD AROUND THE NHS

The website www.nhs.uk has more information on it than you could read in a life-time, but it is the first place to explore to find out about the NHS structure in England, your rights and responsibilities and how to exercise them. In Scotland, go to www.nhsinform.co.uk, in Wales it's www.wales. nhs.uk and in Ireland, it's www.hscni.net. The four countries have four very different systems driven by different ideologies but are all striving to provide treatment according to need. Unfortunately, as with all Western countries, there is a lot of unmet need in all these systems. A lot of money is wasted on expensive bureaucracies, reorganization, marketization, duplication, litigation and tests and treatments of marginal benefit, when what many patients need most is hands-on care that works, and the support to care for themselves. What's clear from the finances of the NHS is that – although it aims to be universal – it can't meet everyone's needs. Complex care costs a lot and requires compassion, competence, collaboration, communication and courage. These are all two-way streets. The best health service in the world doesn't exist – each has its strengths and weaknesses. But for the NHS to survive we need to do far more than fund it, we need to live well outside it and participate inside it.

In England, Healthwatch (www.healthwatch.co.uk) aims to be 'the consumer champion in health and care' – you will find out how useful it is by using your local branch. The Patients Association (www.patients-association.com) is another source of help and support in navigating the NHS. National Voices (www.nationalvoices.org.uk) is a coalition of health and social care charities in England. It aims to strengthen the voice of patients, service users, carers, their families and the voluntary organizations that work for them.

When I trained as a GP, the big idea was that doctors should move from being gods to being guides. Patients would become partners in their care, and technology would help us to move from deciding for you to deciding with you, and then helping you to do as much as you can for yourself. Technology at its best is brilliant at joining up care, creating more time for face to face consultations, supporting better decisions and shifting the balance of power to patients. But it has to be used wisely.

There is already the technology for you to do 200 blood tests on a tiny sample of blood in your home, and have them quickly and accurately analysed. There are contact lenses that continuously monitor the blood sugar of diabetics. You can have all your medical records implanted in a chip under your skin. Wearable devices can monitor your heart rate and rhythm, oxygen saturation, blood pressure, respiratory rate and temperature in real time, all the time, and transmit the data to your mobile phone and beyond to whoever you wish to share it with. Computerised algorithms can analyse your data and tell you when to seek help. All this is already happening. The questions remain; Do you want to know all this data about you? Will it make you more or less anxious? Will it improve your health and healthcare? Will you still be able to find a wise health professional to help you make sense of it? The answers can only come from properly constructed clinical trials. In general, the sicker you are, the more you are helped by accurate, real time data. But if you feel great, data anxiety can ruin you one wild and precious life.

There has never been a more exciting time to participate in medical research – with the sequencing of 100,000 human genomes (www.genomicsengland.co.uk) and the chance for medicine to be personalized to individuals. The questions remain: how well will it work and how much are we prepared to pay for it?

Should our NHS money got towards humane care for the elderly or pushing the boundaries of high tech science to treat conditions that were previously untreatable? Should we dive deeper and deeper into the river of illness to rescue people who are sicker and sicker? Or should we wander upstream and try to stop them falling in? We can only have both if we pay a lot more. At present, NHS hospitals are plunging into debt because they only get paid a third of what their emergency admissions cost them, and they lose over £80,000 for every critically ill patient that costs over £100,000 to treat. There simply isn't enough money in the system to do everything, as the NHS pretends to do. You can't access care if it isn't there. And and the big danger of pretending to be able to do everything without adequate resources is that we become overstretched and dangerous, and end up with more scandals. Time for politicians and NHS staff to have an honest conversation with us about what the NHS is for, and what it could – and should – do with its limited resources. One thing is for sure. No drug can replace living and working with joy and purpose in a kind and connected community. Keep CLANGing.

Keep in touch. And good luck
@drphilhammond

THANKS

The biggest thanks goes to all those who publicly share their stories – some extremely personal and heart-breaking – to help others. You are my leaders. Thanks to Wendy Lee for her generous support and foreword, and David Grant for his helpful feedback.

Thank you to Jenny Heller, formerly of Quercus, for asking me to write this book, and to Richard Milner for picking up the pieces. It's very rare that a publisher asks you to write anything, unless you happen to be terribly famous, so of course I said yes. I then got stuck for months trying not to repeat the previous mistakes I've made telling patients how to be patients. My 'aha' moment came when I realized I needed to do what the NHS needs to do. Listen to patients.

Thanks to Esther Crawley and her brilliant team for giving me a job, supporting me and helping me rediscover the joy of working in the NHS.

And thanks to Jo, Will, Ellie, Mum, Dad, Steve and Stan for all the CLANGERS. You know where they're hidden.

INDEX